AF870186

Pharmacology

for Technicians

Fifth Edition

Instructor's Guide

Don A. Ballington • Mary M. Laughlin

Paradigm PUBLISHING
St. Paul

Managing Editor: Brenda M. Palo
Developmental Editor: Stephanie Schempp and Susan Foster
Production Editor: Sarah Kearin and Lori Michelle Ryan
Cover and Text Designers: Jaana Bykonich and Timothy W. Larson

Care has been taken to verify the accuracy of information presented in this book. However, the authors, editors, and publisher cannot accept responsibility for Web, e-mail, newsgroup, or chat room subject matter or content, or for consequences from application of the information in this book, and make no warranty, expressed or implied, with respect to its content.

Trademarks: Some of the product names and company names included in this book have been used for identification purposes only and may be trademarks or registered trade names of their respective manufacturers and sellers. The authors, editors, and publisher disclaim any affiliation, association, or connection with, or sponsorship or endorsement by, such owners.

We have made every effort to trace the ownership of all copyrighted material and to secure permission from copyright holders. In the event of any question arising as to the use of any material, we will be pleased to make the necessary corrections in future printings. Thanks are due to the aforementioned authors, publishers, and agents for permission to use the materials indicated.

ISBN: 978-0-76385-235-1 (text and Instructor Resources DVD package)
ISBN: 978-0-76385-231-3 (text)

© 2013 Paradigm Publishing, Inc., a division of EMC Publishing, LLC
875 Montreal Way
St. Paul, MN 55102
E-mail: educate@emcp.com
Web site: www.emcp.com

All rights reserved. No part of this publication may be adapted, reproduced, stored in a retrieval system, or transmitted in any form or by any means, electronic, mechanical, photocopying, recording, or otherwise, without prior written permission from the publisher.

Printed in the United States of America

22 21 20 19 18 17 16 15 14 13 1 2 3 4 5 6 7 8 9 10

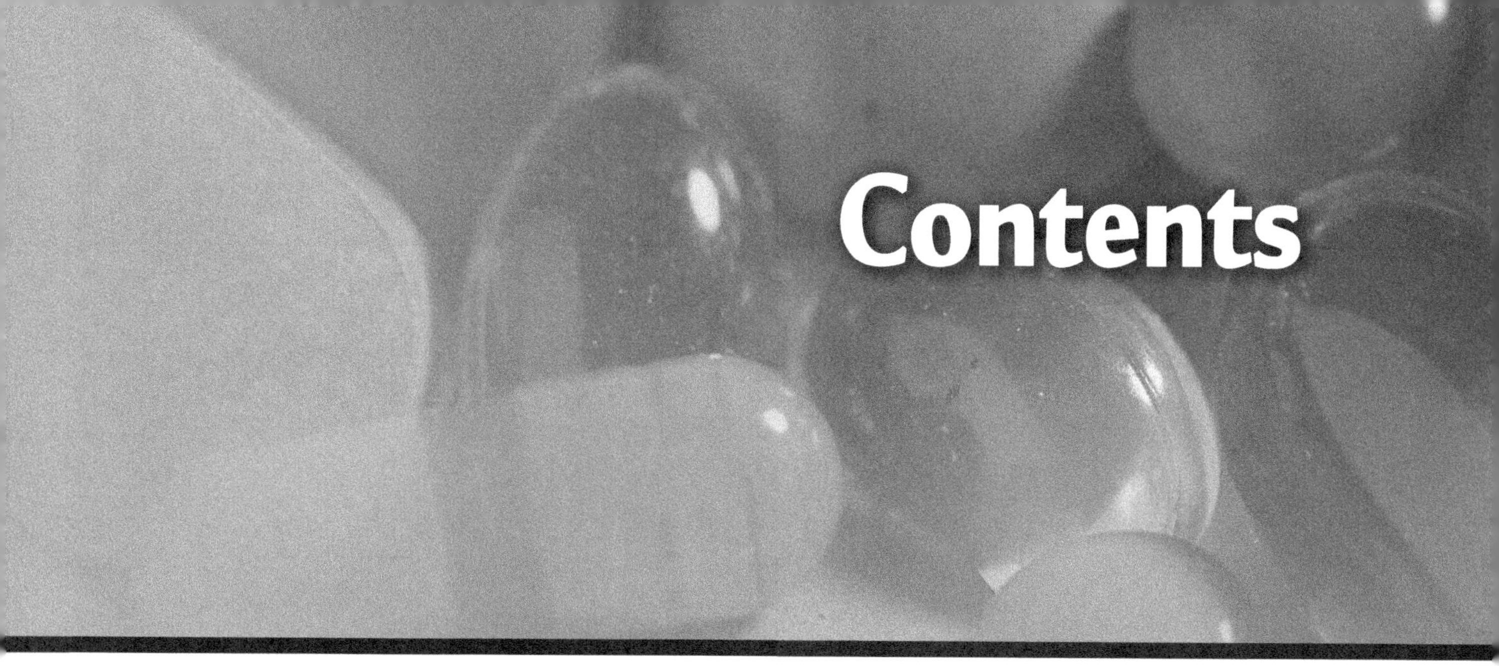

Contents

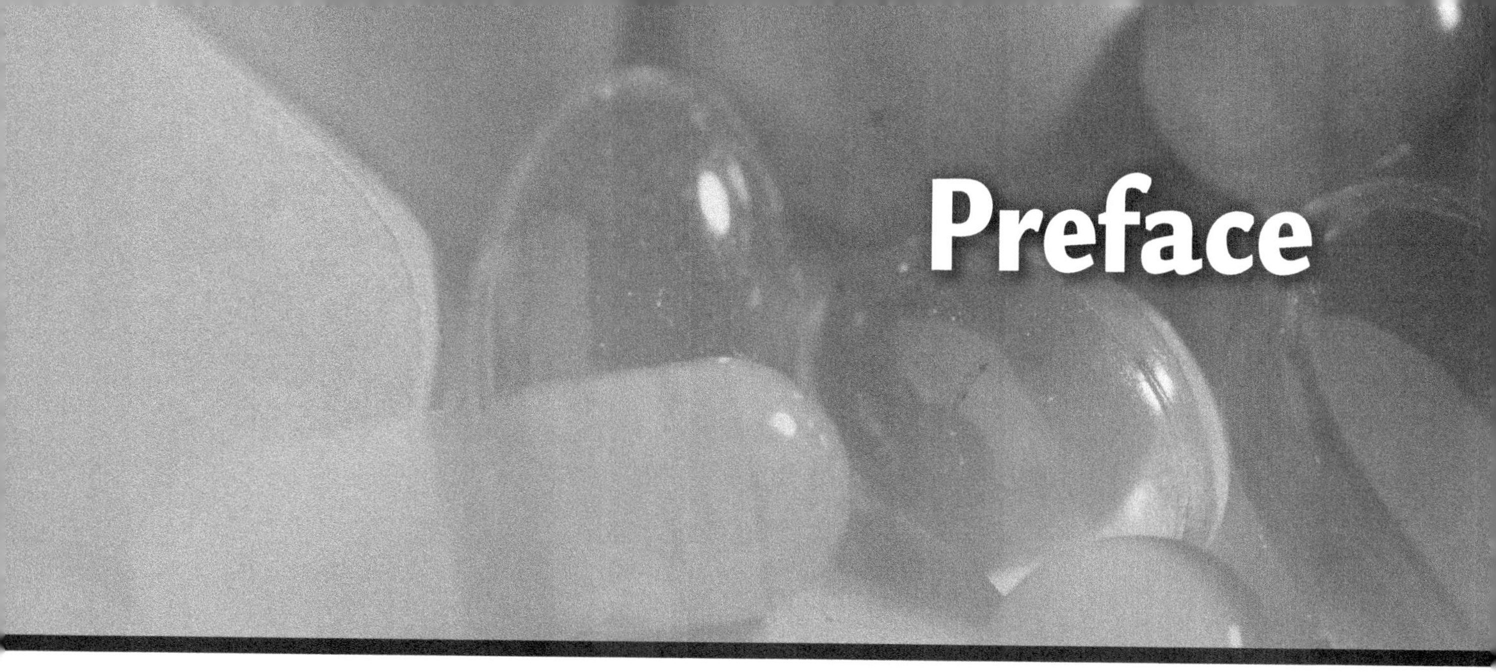

Preface

This Instructor's Guide has been prepared for instructors who are using *Pharmacology for Technicians, Fifth Edition* by Don Ballington and Mary M. Laughlin. This resource will help you plan a comprehensive pharmacology course that allows students to acquire the drug knowledge to satisfy certification requirements and to secure employment as a pharmacy technician.

This Instructor's Guide includes suggested course objectives to help you plan course content and model syllabi to help with course structure and assignments. For each chapter, there are teaching hints as well as answers to the end-of-chapter questions. Answers to all exercises in the *Pharmacology for Technicians Workbook, Fifth Edition*, are also included. The Instructor's Guide includes quizzes for each chapter, tests for each of the four units, a midterm exam for Chapters 1–9 and another midterm exam for Chapters 10–17, and a final exam that covers the entire book. This resource concludes with answers to all of the exercises included in the workbook.

Many of the items included in this Instructor's Guide are also available on the DVD that accompanies this guide as well as on the password-protected instructor's section of the Internet Resource Center (website) for this title at www.paradigmcollege.net/pharmacology5e. The DVD and website also contain PowerPoint slides. Additional information for both students and instructors is available within the Preface of *Pharmacology for Technicians, Fifth Edition.*

The authors and editorial staff encourage your feedback on the text and its supplements. Please reach us by clicking the "Contact Us" button at www.emcp.com.

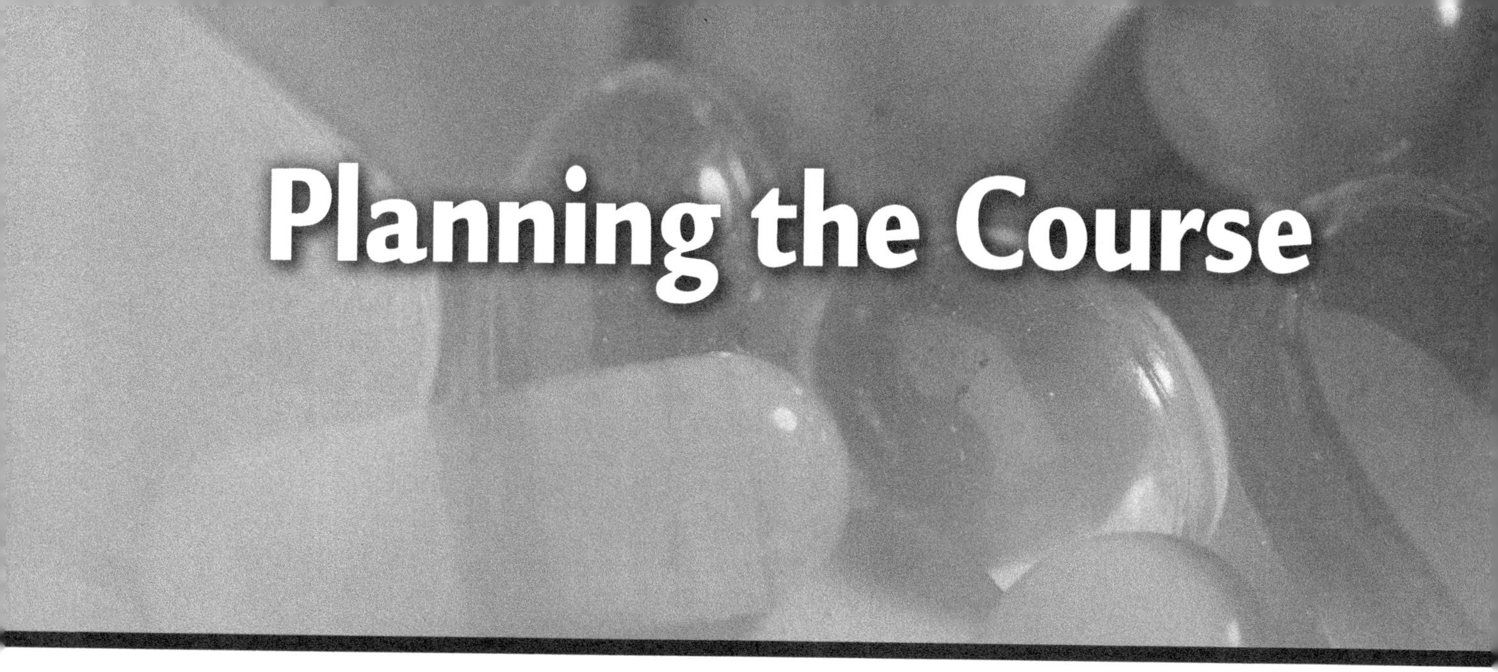

Planning the Course

Most educators would agree that the key to teaching a successful course is careful, thorough planning. And, as noted in *Exceptional Teaching: Ideas in Action*, published by Paradigm Publishing, "Instructors assess, plan, implement, and evaluate . . . repeatedly. They do this based on many of the factors that make teaching learner-centered and on several other variables. Before students even think about entering or logging into the classroom, instructors make decisions about the course. These begin with identifying the heart of the course. That is, what, exactly, are the most important objectives and course outcomes? And what plan of action can the instructor devise that will help ensure those outcomes?" Thinking through a course action plan typically includes four phases:

1. Developing the course outcomes
2. Determining the course delivery mode and structure (dividing the course into parts, each with outcomes)
3. Selecting the course's instructional approach, resources, and activities
4. Developing an assessment strategy

Developing Course Goals

In developing course outcomes, some of the key issues to consider are the following:

- When this course is over, in what ways will the learner be permanently changed? Should instruction result in
    - building knowledge?
    - developing higher-order thinking?
    - developing independent learning skills?
    - developing technical literacy?
- Think about the course content in terms of what types of problems are faced.
    - What decisions are made?
    - What must be communicated?
    - Under what conditions is the work performed on the job?
    - How will the performer learn the work is satisfactory?
    - How will the performer receive feedback?

Considering the questions above, a set of course objectives could include the following items:

1. Examine principles of drug action in the body and individual cells, including body absorption and distribution in relation to therapeutic blood levels and the process of clearing systemically dispersed agents through metabolism and elimination.
2. Anticipate how best to promote safety and avoid medication errors through drug label and medication order literacy skills. Be able to communicate effectively with patients and other members of the healthcare team. Implement appropriate patient warning labels to promote thorough understanding of drug regimen requirements by patients and medical staff.
3. Anticipate possible side effects and related dispensing strategy for each drug class as well as for specific agents. Analyze labeling requirements for various classes of pharmaceuticals and cautions when dispensing based on thorough understanding of interactions between classes of pharmaceuticals, individual agents, and natural supplements.
4. Describe ways various classes of anti-infective drugs work against microorganisms and identify uses of these drugs in eliminating specific microorganisms from the body.
5. Explain the action of neurotransmitters in the nervous system, relate classes of pharmaceuticals that affect or change neurotransmitter action, and describe therapeutic results obtained with the various neurological agent classes.
6. Explain principles of how various classes of pharmaceuticals act when utilized in aiding respiratory gas exchanges, circulating blood pressure and cardiac rhythms, and blood filtration.
7. Compare action of pharmaceutical agents when applied to the digestive system and examine, compare, and describe how these agents affect other physiological processes (e.g., blood pressure and sugar levels).
8. Define the action of the endocrine glands and hormones, delineate hormone supplement and replacement therapies, and compile adverse effects of inadequate and excess administration.
9. Identify the physiological action and deficiency symptoms of vitamin classes, explore natural supplements and potential therapeutic value, and examine the use of natural supplements in conjunction with prescription medications.

Determining the Course Delivery Mode and Structure

Whether you are planning a traditional on-campus course, an online or distance learning course, or a hybrid of the two, the core considerations are the same. Chief among them are the course outcomes, class schedule, student characteristics, course subject matter, and available resources. The instructional delivery differences among the delivery modes, however, create distinct needs you must address in the planning stage. Because online and hybrid courses represent a minority of college classes—although a growing minority—they offer special challenges for instructors, particularly educators new to these delivery modes.

Online and Hybrid Courses: Special Considerations

A critical challenge in teaching online courses is the issue of interacting with the students. How will you communicate with them? How will they submit assignments and tests? How will you deliver feedback? How will you get to know your students?

Here are some additional questions to consider when planning an online or hybrid course, as suggested in *Exceptional Teaching:*

1. What course management system will be used: Blackboard, WebCT, or some other platform?
2. Will you offer a Web course where everything is done online? Or, will you teach a course where students work independently offline and use the course management system to review course outcomes, the syllabus, assignment due dates; communicate with the instructor; take online quizzes; transmit completed work; and participate in chat sessions?
3. Will you have an on-campus orientation meeting with your students at the beginning of the course? In some situations, because of the distance factor, students will not be able to come to campus. However, if feasible, by all means do so. Many students will likely have the same questions that can be answered at one time, and the face-to-face contact at an orientation will benefit both you and the students.
4. Will the students come to the campus or school to take exams? If not, will students be directed to offsite locations where exams can be administered to verify that the person taking the exam is indeed the person getting credit for the course? It is critical that this step be set up before the online class begins.
5. What PC configuration and/or software requirements must a student have to participate in your online course?

Both the student and instructor resources offered with *Pharmacology for Technicians, Fifth Edition* can be adapted for online learning or a hybrid of traditional and online learning contexts. Certain product components have been developed specifically for these environments. A Class Connection pre-built Learning Management System (LMS) cartridge is available with pre-loaded resources, and the ExamView Assessment Suite makes it easy to develop quizzes and tests and deliver them on the Web. These supplements are discussed in more detail in the subsection titled *Selecting the Instructional Approach, Resources, and Activities.*

Course Structure and Syllabus

Textbook authors typically design their content to align with the most popular course structure for a particular subject, and they develop syllabus plans that correlate with that framework. In this situation, much of your basic planning is therefore completed, and you may only need to modify the course structure and the resulting syllabus slightly. If you are in a position to develop a plan or modify an existing structure, consider these questions:

- What topics are essential for demonstrating the course outcomes?
- Is this the only course that will address this subject and skill set?
- What do students already know about the subject, its subtopics, and its associated skill set? What can they learn on their own independently of your direct instruction?
- Where in each topic will the instruction "begin" and "end"?

A comprehensive syllabus should help you and your students prepare for each part of the class. Syllabi are useful for both traditional on-campus courses as well as courses that are delivered online. Generally, the following elements are included in a syllabus:

1. Course identifying data
2. Prerequisites
3. Instructor contact information
4. Course objectives
5. Required course resources
6. Major assignments
7. Grade composition
8. Class structure
9. Course schedule
10. College/school requirements

The following sample syllabi are presented: (1) Syllabus I is an example of a traditional on-campus course syllabus designed for a one-semester, 16-week course that meets three times a week using *Pharmacology for Technicians, Fifth Edition*. (2) Syllabus 2 is an example of a syllabus for a two-semester, 32-week course using *Pharmacology for Technicians, Fifth Edition*. (3) Syllabus 3 is a syllabus for a quarter-based course that consists of two 10-week sessions. (4) Syllabus 4 shows a syllabus for four 5-week modules. Word documents for each of these syllabus suggestions are available on the Instructor Resources disc and for download from the password-protected instructor side of the Internet Resource Center for this textbook at www.paradigmcollege.net/pharmacology5e. You can use these documents as a starting point for your own course syllabus.

Syllabus I: 16-Week Semester

Course Description

This course introduces pharmacy technician students to the general principles of pharmacology. Drugs are discussed in the context of drug classes, mechanics of action, disease types, and body systems. The goal is to provide pharmacy technicians with sufficient background information so that they will be able to play a key role in avoiding dispensing errors. Although emphasis will be given to the approximately 200 most commonly prescribed drugs, many more drugs will be discussed during the semester.

Prerequisites: [Depends on specific pharmacy technician program]

Instructor Contact Information

Name:
Office Phone:
Office E-mail:
Office Location:
Office Hours:

Required Course Resources

Pharmacology for Technicians, Fifth Edition with Study Partner CD and Pocket Guide for Technicians

Pharmacology for Technicians Workbook, Fifth Edition [Decision to assign Workbook is up to individual instructor or pharmacy technician program]

www.paradigmcollege.net/pharmacology5e

Study Time

Approximately six to eight hours per week of study or homework time outside of class is recommended for successful completion of course requirements.

Grading

Final grades will be calculated as follows:

Attendance	5%
Homework, including Study Partner Reported Mode quizzes, Workbook	30%
Team reports	10%
Chapter quizzes	10%
Midterm exams	25%
Final exam	20%

College and Course Policy Information

- This college conforms to the provisions of the Americans with Disabilities Act. You are invited to report any special needs to your instructor.
- Your attendance is expected at all class sessions. Excessive unexcused absences may result in dismissal from the class.
- Cell phone use (ringing, answering, text messaging) is not allowed in class.
- We subscribe to the college policy on academic honesty found in the school catalog.

Course Schedule

Week	Session	Text Reference	Assessments	Workbook Assignment Due*
1	1	Chapter 1		
	2	Chapter 1	Chapter 1 Quiz	
	3	Chapter 2		Chapter 1
2	4	Chapter 2	Chapter 2 Quiz	
	5	Chapter 3		Chapter 2
	6	Chapter 3	Chapter 3 Quiz	
3	7	Chapter 4		Chapter 3
	8	Chapter 4		
	9	Chapter 4	Chapter 4 Quiz	
4	10	Chapter 5		Chapter 4
	11	Chapter 5		
	12		Midterm Exam covering Chapters 1–5	Chapter 5
5	13	Chapter 6		
	14	Chapter 6		
	15	Chapter 6	Chapter 6 Quiz	
6	16	Chapter 7		Chapter 6
	17	Chapter 7	Chapter 7 Quiz	
	18	Chapter 8		Chapter 7
7	19	Chapter 8	Chapter 8 Quiz	
	20	Chapter 9		Chapter 8
	21	Chapter 9		
8	22	Chapter 9		
	23		Midterm Exam covering Chapters 6–9	Chapter 9
	24	Chapter 10		
9	25	Chapter 10		
	26	Chapter 10	Chapter 10 Quiz	
	27	Chapter 11		Chapter 10

Week	Session	Text Reference	Assessments	Workbook Assignment Due*
10	28 29 30	Chapter 11 Chapter 12 Chapter 12	Chapter 11 Quiz	Chapter 11
11	31 32 33	Chapter 12 Chapter 13 Chapter 13	Chapter 12 Quiz Chapter 13 Quiz	Chapter 12
12	34 35 36	Chapter 14 Chapter 14 Chapter 14		Chapter 13
13	37 38 39	 Chapter 15 Chapter 15	Midterm Exam covering Chapters 10–14	Chapter 14
14	40 41 42	Chapter 15 Chapter 16 Chapter 16	Chapter 15 Quiz	Chapter 15
15	43 44 45	Chapter 16 Chapter 17 Chapter 17	Chapter 16 Quiz Chapter 17 Quiz	Chapter 16
16	46 47 48	Review for Final Exam Review for Final Exam	 Final Exam	Chapter 17

*Only applicable if Workbook is assigned

Syllabus 2: Two Semesters

Course Description

This course introduces pharmacy technician students to the general principles of pharmacology. Drugs are discussed in the context of drug classes, mechanics of action, disease types, and body systems. The goal is to provide pharmacy technicians with sufficient background information so that they will be able to play a key role in avoiding dispensing errors. Although emphasis will be given to the approximately 200 most commonly prescribed drugs, many more drugs will be discussed during the semester.

Prerequisites: [Depends on specific pharmacy technician program]

Instructor Contact Information

Name:
Office Phone:
Office E-mail:
Office Location:
Office Hours:

Required Course Resources

Pharmacology for Technicians, Fifth Edition with Study Partner CD and Pocket Guide for Technicians

Pharmacology for Technicians Workbook, Fifth Edition [Decision to assign Workbook is up to individual instructor or pharmacy technician program]

www.paradigmcollege.net/pharmacology5e

Study Time

Approximately six to eight hours per week of study or homework time outside of class is recommended for successful completion of course requirements.

Grading

Final grades will be calculated as follows:

Attendance	5%
Homework, including Study Partner Reported Mode quizzes, Workbook	30%
Team reports	10%
Chapter quizzes	10%
Midterm exams	25%
Final exam	20%

College and Course Policy Information

- This college conforms to the provisions of the Americans with Disabilities Act. You are invited to report any special needs to your instructor.
- Your attendance is expected at all class sessions. Excessive unexcused absences may result in dismissal from the class.
- Cell phone use (ringing, answering, text messaging) is not allowed in class.
- We subscribe to the college policy on academic honesty found in the school catalog.

Course Schedule

Semester 1

Week	Session	Text Reference	Assessments	Workbook Assignment Due*
1	1	Chapter 1		
	2	Chapter 1		
	3	Chapter 1	Chapter 1 Quiz	
2	4	Chapter 2		Chapter 1
	5	Chapter 2		
	6	Chapter 2	Chapter 2 Quiz	
3	7	Chapter 2		
	8	Chapter 3		Chapter 2
	9	Chapter 3		
4	10	Chapter 3		
	11	Chapter 3		
	12	Chapters 1–3 Review		Chapter 3
5	13		Midterm Exam covering Chapters 1–3	
	14	Chapter 4		
	15	Chapter 4		
6	16	Chapter 4		
	17	Chapter 4		
	18	Chapter 4		
7	19	Chapter 4		
	20	Chapter 4	Chapter 4 Quiz	
	21	Chapter 5		Chapter 4
8	22	Chapter 5		
	23	Chapter 5		
	24	Chapter 5	Chapter 5 Quiz	

Week	Session	Text Reference	Assessments	Workbook Assignment Due*
9	25 26 27	Chapter 6 Chapter 6 Chapter 6		Chapter 5
10	28 29 30	Chapter 6 Chapter 6 Chapter 6		
11	31 32 33	Chapters 4–6 Review Chapter 7	 Midterm Exam covering Chapters 4–6	Chapter 6
12	34 35 36	Chapter 7 Chapter 7 Chapter 7	 Chapter 7 Quiz	
13	37 38 39	Chapter 8 Chapter 8 Chapter 8		Chapter 7
14	40 41 42	Chapter 8 Chapter 9 Chapter 9	Chapter 8 Quiz	 Chapter 8
15	43 44 45	Chapter 9 Chapter 9 Chapter 9		
16	46 47 48	Review for Final Exam Review for Final Exam	 Final Exam	Chapter 9

*Only applicable if Workbook is assigned

Semester 2

Week	Session	Text Reference	Assessments	Workbook Assignment Due*
1	1 2 3	Chapter 10 Chapter 10 Chapter 10		
2	4 5 6	Chapter 10 Chapter 10 Chapter 10	 Chapter 10 Quiz	
3	7 8 9	Chapter 11 Chapter 11 Chapter 11		Chapter 10
4	10 11	Chapter 11 Chapters 10 & 11 Review		 Chapter 11
	12		Midterm Exam covering Chapters 10–11	

Week	Session	Text Reference	Assessments	Workbook Assignment Due*
5	13	Chapter 12		
	14	Chapter 12		
	15	Chapter 12		
6	16	Chapter 12		
	17	Chapter 12		
	18	Chapter 12		
7	19	Chapter 12	Chapter 12 Quiz	
	20	Chapter 13		Chapter 12
	21	Chapter 13		
8	22	Chapter 13	Chapter 13 Quiz	
	23	Chapter 14		Chapter 13
	24	Chapter 14		
9	25	Chapter 14		
	26	Chapter 14		
	27	Chapter 14		
10	28	Chapter 14		
	29	Chapter 14	Chapter 14 Quiz	
	30	Chapter 13 & 14 Review		Chapter 14
11	31		Midterm Exam covering Chapters 13–14	
	32	Chapter 15		
	33	Chapter 15		
12	34	Chapter 15		
	35	Chapter 15		
	36	Chapter 15	Chapter 15 Quiz	
13	37	Chapter 16		Chapter 15
	38	Chapter 16		
	39	Chapter 16		
14	40	Chapter 16		
	41	Chapter 16	Chapter 16 Quiz	Chapter 16
	42	Chapter 17		
15	43	Chapter 17		
	44	Chapter 17		
	45	Chapter 17		
16	46	Review for Final Exam		Chapter 17
	47	Review for Final Exam		
	48		Final Exam	

*Only applicable if Workbook is assigned

Syllabus 3: Two 10-Week Quarters

Course Description

This course introduces pharmacy technician students to the general principles of pharmacology. Drugs are discussed in the context of drug classes, mechanics of action, disease types, and body systems. The goal is to provide pharmacy technicians with sufficient background information so that they will be able to play a key role in avoiding dispensing errors. Although emphasis will be given to the approximately 200 most commonly prescribed drugs, many more drugs will be discussed during the semester.

Prerequisites: [Depends on specific pharmacy technician program]

Instructor Contact Information

Name:
Office Phone:
Office E-mail:
Office Location:
Office Hours:

Required Course Resources

Pharmacology for Technicians, Fifth Edition with Study Partner CD and *Pocket Guide for Technicians*

Pharmacology for Technicians Workbook, Fifth Edition [Decision to assign Workbook is up to individual instructor or pharmacy technician program]

www.paradigmcollege.net/pharmacology5e

Study Time

Approximately six to eight hours per week of study or homework time outside of class is recommended for successful completion of course requirements.

Grading

Final grades will be calculated as follows:

Attendance	5%
Homework, including Study Partner Reported Mode quizzes, Workbook	30%
Team reports	10%
Chapter quizzes	10%
Midterm exams	25%
Final exam	20%

College and Course Policy Information

- This college conforms to the provisions of the Americans with Disabilities Act. You are invited to report any special needs to your instructor.
- Your attendance is expected at all class sessions. Excessive unexcused absences may result in dismissal from the class.
- Cell phone use (ringing, answering, text messaging) is not allowed in class.
- We subscribe to the college policy on academic honesty found in the school catalog.

Course Schedule

Quarter 1

Week	Session	Text Reference	Assessments	Workbook Assignment Due*
1	1	Chapter 1		
	2	Chapter 1	Chapter 1 Quiz	
	3	Chapter 2		Chapter 1
2	4	Chapter 2	Chapter 2 Quiz	
	5	Chapter 3		Chapter 2
	6	Chapter 3	Chapter 3 Quiz	
3	7	Chapter 4		Chapter 3
	8	Chapter 4		
	9	Chapter 4		Chapter 4
4	10		Midterm Exam covering Chapters 1–4	
	11	Chapter 5		
	12	Chapter 5		
5	13	Chapter 5	Chapter 5 Quiz	
	14	Chapter 6		Chapter 5
	15	Chapter 6		
6	16	Chapter 6		
	17	Chapter 6	Chapter 6 Quiz	
	18	Chapter 7		Chapter 6
7	19	Chapter 7		
	20	Chapter 7		Chapter 7
	21		Midterm Exam covering Chapters 5–7	
8	22	Chapter 8		
	23	Chapter 8		
	24	Chapter 8	Chapter 8 Quiz	
9	25	Chapter 9		Chapter 8
	26	Chapter 9		
	27	Chapter 9		
10	28	Chapter 9		
	29	Final Exam Review		Chapter 9
	30		Final	

*Only applicable if Workbook is assigned

Quarter 2

Week	Session	Text Reference	Assessments	Workbook Assignment Due*
1	1	Chapter 10		
	2	Chapter 10		
	3	Chapter 10		
2	4	Chapter 10	Chapter 10 Quiz	
	5	Chapter 11		Chapter 10
	6	Chapter 11	Chapter 11 Quiz	
3	7	Chapter 12		Chapter 11
	8	Chapter 12		
	9	Chapter 12		
4	10	Chapter 12	Chapter 12 Quiz	Chapter 12
	11		Midterm Exam covering Chapters 10–12	
	12	Chapter 13		
5	13	Chapter 13	Chapter 13 Quiz	
	14	Chapter 14		Chapter 13
	15	Chapter 14		
6	16	Chapter 14		
	17	Chapter 14		
	18	Chapter 14		Chapter 14
7	19		Midterm Exam covering Chapters 13–14	
	20	Chapter 15		
	21	Chapter 15		
8	22	Chapter 15	Chapter 15 Quiz	
	23	Chapter 16		Chapter 15
	24	Chapter 16		
9	25	Chapter 16	Chapter 16 Quiz	
	26	Chapter 17		Chapter 16
	27	Chapter 17		
10	28	Chapter 17		
	29	Final Exam Review		Chapter 17
	30		Final Exam	

*Only applicable if Workbook is assigned

Syllabus 4: Four 5-Week Modules

Course Description

This course introduces pharmacy technician students to the general principles of pharmacology. Drugs are discussed in the context of drug classes, mechanics of action, disease types, and body systems. The goal is to provide pharmacy technicians with sufficient background information so that they will be able to play a key role in avoiding dispensing errors. Although emphasis will be given to the approximately 200 most commonly prescribed drugs, many more drugs will be discussed during the semester.

Prerequisites: [Depends on specific pharmacy technician program]

Instructor Contact Information

Name:
Office Phone:
Office E-mail:
Office Location:
Office Hours:

Required Course Resources

Pharmacology for Technicians, Fifth Edition with Study Partner CD and *Pocket Guide for Technicians*

Pharmacology for Technicians Workbook, Fifth Edition [Decision to assign Workbook is up to individual instructor or pharmacy technician program]

www.paradigmcollege.net/pharmacology5e

Study Time

Approximately six to eight hours per week of study or homework time outside of class is recommended for successful completion of course requirements.

Grading

Final grades will be calculated as follows:

Attendance	5%
Homework, including Study Partner Reported quizzes, Workbook	30%
Team reports	10%
Chapter quizzes	10%
Midterm exams	20%
Final exam	25%

College and Course Policy Information

- This college conforms to the provisions of the Americans with Disabilities Act. You are invited to report any special needs to your instructor.
- Your attendance is expected at all class sessions. Excessive unexcused absences may result in dismissal from the class.
- Cell phone use (ringing, answering, text messaging) is not allowed in class.
- We subscribe to the college policy on academic honesty found in the school catalog.

Course Schedule

Module 1

Week	Session	Text Reference	Assessments	Workbook Assignment Due*
1	1	Chapter 1		
	2	Chapter 1	Chapter 1 Quiz	
	3	Chapter 2		Chapter 1
	4	Chapter 2	Chapter 2 Quiz	
2	5	Chapter 3		Chapter 2
	6	Chapter 3		
	7	Chapter 3		
	8	Review Chapters 1–3		Chapter 3
3	9		Mid-module exam covering Chapters 1–3	
	10	Chapter 4		
	11	Chapter 4		
	12	Chapter 4		
4	13	Chapter 4		
	14	Chapter 4	Chapter 4 Quiz	
	15	Chapter 5		Chapter 4
	16	Chapter 5		
5	17	Chapter 5		
	18	Chapter 5		
	19	Final Exam Review		Chapter 5
	20		Module 1 Final Exam covering chapters 1–5	

*Only applicable if Workbook is assigned

Module 2

Week	Session	Text Reference	Assessments	Workbook Assignment Due*
1	1	Chapter 6		
	2	Chapter 6		
	3	Chapter 6		
	4	Chapter 6	Chapter 6 Quiz	
2	5	Chapter 7		Chapter 6
	6	Chapter 7		
	7	Chapter 7		
	8	Chapter 7		
3	9	Review Chapters 6–7		Chapter 7
	10		Mid-module exam covering Chapters 6–7	
	11	Chapter 8		
	12	Chapter 8		
4	13	Chapter 8	Chapter 8 Quiz	
	14	Chapter 9		Chapter 8
	15	Chapter 9		
	16	Chapter 9		

Week	Session	Text Reference	Assessments	Workbook Assignment Due*
5	17	Chapter 9		
	18	Chapter 9		
	19	Final Exam Review		Chapter 9
	20		Module 2 Final Exam covering chapters 6–9	

*Only applicable if Workbook is assigned

Module 3

Week	Session	Text Reference	Assessments	Workbook Assignment Due*
1	1	Chapter 10		
	2	Chapter 10		
	3	Chapter 10		
	4	Chapter 10	Chapter 10 Quiz	
2	5	Chapter 11		Chapter 10
	6	Chapter 11		
	7	Chapter 11		
	8	Chapter 11		
3	9	Review Chapters 10–11		Chapter 11
	10		Mid-module exam covering Chapters 10–11	
	11	Chapter 12		
	12	Chapter 12		
4	13	Chapter 12		
	14	Chapter 12		
	15	Chapter 12	Chapter 12 Quiz	
	16	Chapter 13		Chapter 12
5	17	Chapter 13		
	18	Chapter 13		
	19	Final Exam Review		Chapter 13
	20		Module 3 Final Exam covering chapters 10–13	

*Only applicable if Workbook is assigned

Module 4

Week	Session	Text Reference	Assessments	Workbook Assignment Due*
1	1	Chapter 14		
	2	Chapter 14		
	3	Chapter 14		
	4	Chapter 14		
2	5	Chapter 14	Chapter 14 Quiz	
	6	Chapter 15		Chapter 14
	7	Chapter 15		
	8	Chapter 15		
3	9	Chapter 15		
	10	Review Chapters 14–15		Chapter 15
	11		Mid-module exam covering Chapters 14–15	
	12	Chapter 16		
4	13	Chapter 16		
	14	Chapter 16		
	15	Chapter 16	Chapter 16 Quiz	
	16	Chapter 17		Chapter 16
5	17	Chapter 17		
	18	Chapter 17		
	19	Final Exam Review		Chapter 17
	20		Module 4 Final Exam covering Chapters 14–17	

Selecting the Instructional Approach, Resources, and Activities

After the course outcomes, delivery mode, and structure are determined, it is important to plan the main content of the course. This includes selecting courseware, identifying resources for English-language learners, considering instructional support materials, and reviewing supplemental resources.

Student Courseware

Selecting high-quality student courseware is an important step in the planning process. Learning materials should be engaging and accessible. Paradigm Publishing's Pharmacology for Technicians product includes several valuable learning tools to support the course performance objectives.

- *Pharmacology for Technicians, Fifth Edition*
- Study Partner CD
- Student Internet Resource Center at www.paradigmcollege.net/pharmacology5e
- *Pharmacology for Technicians Workbook, Fifth Edition*

Textbook Structure

Pharmacology for Technicians, Fifth Edition is designed to help students learn the basic principles of pharmacology and to become familiar with the most commonly prescribed drugs. Key features of the text include the following:

- **Learning Objectives** at the beginning of each chapter establish clear goals and focus chapter study.
- **Key Terms** are shown in boldface and defined in context, where they first appear in the text discussion. Students are encouraged to preview the chapter terms on the Study Partner CD at the start of each chapter. Chapter terms are also listed at the conclusion of each chapter for quick reference. A complete glossary appears at the back of the book. Another tool for learning the language of pharmacology is the Study Partner CD, which provides audio of all of the chapter terms and definitions plus flash cards.
- **Overview Discussions** of the anatomy and physiology of the featured body system of each chapter and the pathology of the diseases that affect that system are provided.
- **Photos and Figures** visually reinforce the information taught in the chapter.
- **Drug Tables** provide generic and brand names for more than 1,000 drugs. Also, for these drugs the tables include a pronunciation guide for generic names, dosage forms, dispensing status, and for some drugs the controlled-substance schedule.
- **Warning Stickers** in margins provide examples of the types of information pharmacy technician students will share with patients.
- **Warning Sidebars** point out potential points of confusion, such as drug names that are spelled alike and pills that look alike.
- **Chapter Terms** at the back of each chapter list the important terminology, with definitions.
- **Chapter Summary** provides an overview of the key points of the chapter.
- **Drug List** at the back of chapters 4–17 provides a comprehensive list of drugs discussed in each chapter, including those drugs that require a medication guide or a black box warning when dispensed.
- **Chapter Review** contains a variety of exercises to help build and assess students' mastery of content.
- **Appendixes** include a list of the most commonly prescribed drugs (A), a list of the top drugs dispensed in hospitals (B), a discussion of look-alike and sound-alike drug names with information on resources to avoid these potential problems (C), and a list of abbreviations used in the book (D).

Study Partner CD

Available with each textbook, the Study Partner CD provides several features to help support student learning.

- Chapter terms and definitions include audio support and an image bank of key illustrations and photographs from the textbook. Terminology review is also supported with flash cards.
- Matching activities reinforce chapter terms and concepts, assess familiarity with generic and brand drug names, and require the student to demonstrate an understanding of chapter content.
- Multiple-choice quizzing in Practice and Reported modes, with feedback, are available for both book and chapter levels.

Pharmacology Internet Resource Center

The Pharmacology Internet Resource Center at www.paradigmcollege.net/pharmacology5e offers valuable information for both instructors and students. For students, the Internet Resource Center includes additional information and learning tools. Through the Web Links page, students can visit useful websites. For English-language learners, Spanish for Pharmacy Technicians is also available, under the Pharmacy Library tab.

Resources for instructors are available on the password-protected Instructor site and include all of the electronic materials found on the Instructor Resources CD.

Instructor's Guide

In addition to course planning tools and suggested syllabi, the *Instructor's Guide* provides answers for all of the end-of-chapter exercises, answers to Workbook exercises, and chapter-specific teaching hints. The *Instructor's Guide* also provides ready-to-use chapter quizzes, unit tests, and final examinations.

Instructor Resources CD

Available with each print *Instructor's Guide*, the Instructor Resources CD includes Microsoft® Word documents of all the resources in the print Instructor's Guide as well as PowerPoint® presentations to enhance lectures.

ExamView® Assessment Suite and Test Banks

The test banks for *Pharmacology for Technicians, Fifth Edition* provide 45–50 multiple choice questions for each chapter. If the provided bank of items doesn't perfectly meet your needs, the program allows you to add an unlimited number of your own items or edit existing items. You can select new or existing items to create an unlimited number of chapter quizzes, tests, and exams. Using the Exam*View* program, you can deliver tests on the Web, on your local area network, or in print. Items included on the test bank are not duplicated on the Study Partner CD.

Class Connection

The Class Connection is a pre-built Learning Management System (LMS) cartridge, effective for distance or hybrid learning. Designed to work with your current LMS, the Class Connection allows you to create a customized Web component for your course. The Class Connection is available in an IMS Content Package that is compatible with all the major LMSs. You can manage your course online using the administrative functions for scheduling, the assessment function for evaluating, and the communication tools for e-conferencing. Instructor materials include a syllabus, a bank of test items for each chapter, and teaching and presentation material. Student material includes study aids, self-tests, and Web links.

Online course management systems such as Blackboard, WebCT, Desire 2 Learn, Angel, and others offer similar tools instructors can use in organizing and teaching a class designed to train pharmacy technicians. Here are ideas for using some of the common tools to their best advantage.

- **Discussion Board.** The discussion board provides an opportunity for every student to interact and become an active learner by posting answers to the weekly discussion question and responding to other student postings.
- **Assignment Tool.** The assignment tool provides an opportunity for students to upload their homework assignment and have the instructor grade and return either

a corrected copy of the assignment or post the corrected solution so students can compare their answers to the corrected solution.

- **Voice Streaming.** The latest technology enables the instructor to use voice streaming to introduce each weekly topic and provide additional instruction and guidance to students. Voice streaming can help auditory learners who benefit from both reading the material in the textbook and listening to an instructor's lecture.
- **Chat Room.** Chat rooms can provide a non-synchronized forum for students and can also allow both the instructor and other students to interact in real time.
- **Assessment Tool.** The test bank can be uploaded into the assessment tool so that students can take their quizzes and exams entirely online. One popular technique for creating unique exams is to use the odd-numbered questions from the test bank for creating randomly generated quizzes while saving the even-numbered questions from the test bank for creating randomly generated exams and finals.
- **Web Links.** Online courses also provide an opportunity for students to conduct information searches on the Internet and submit research papers as part of their course grade. The instructor can post links to websites such as the Institute for Safe Medication Practices for students to peruse and then answer questions on some of the latest issues in relation to avoiding medication errors.

Developing an Assessment Strategy

The final major phase of planning a course is to develop an assessment strategy based on the purpose of evaluation and on your philosophy of what constitutes a high-quality assessment. The obvious purpose of assessing students' learning is to determine whether or not students have achieved the goals of the course and, if they have, determining to what degree, resulting in a grade for credits earned. Other functions of evaluation include motivating students, determining the overall effectiveness of your teaching, and meeting accreditation requirements.

What is your philosophy of assessment? In shaping one, consider these suggestions from Paradigm Publishing's *Exceptional Teaching*:

1. Assessment should contribute to students' learning by asking them to apply their skills in out-of-school or workplace situations.
2. Timing, content, and form of assessments should be planned as an integral part of the course design.
3. The purpose of every assessment should be clear.
4. The type of assessment—its content and format—should be appropriate for the purpose.
5. Assessments should be scored as consistently and objectively as possible.
6. Assessments should provide students with feedback on their learning.
7. Assessments should emphasize intellectual traits of value: analytical reading, thinking, decision making, and research skills along with individual creativity and individual intelligence.
8. Assessments should be conducted at specific, planned checkpoints.
9. Assessments should be conducted in a positive learning environment, with every effort made to lower students' test anxieties.

10. Assessments should allow students to demonstrate their accomplishment of outcomes in various ways, including ways that fit their individual learning styles.

Determining the Number, Level, and Type of Assessments

Using your philosophy of assessment as a guide, begin to formulate your evaluation and grading strategy by answering these course-level questions, as presented in *Exceptional Teaching*:

- Do I want a course pre-assessment?
- Do I want a course comprehensive assessment—one that will determine students' mastery of the major intended outcomes for the entire course?
- Do I want pre-assessments for each section or program?
- Do I want comprehensive assessments for each section or program—ones that assess students' mastery of the major intended outcomes for that program?
- Do I want interim or checkpoint assessments that assess students' mastery of intended outcomes of learning chunks within units? How many? How often?
- Once my system is in place, will my students know that I value *how* and *how well* they think?

The questions above will help you establish approximately how many assessments you wish to include and their place in the course. The next decisions concern which types of assessment to use: traditional cognitive (objective) tests and/or performance-based assessments. Each of these two major categories of tests has its best uses. Traditional cognitive tests such as multiple-choice exams usually work best for testing information recall, comprehension, and analysis. They also are reliable and efficient, and relatively easy to score. On the down side, objective-type tests are criticized for not representing how students will use their new skills in an unfamiliar setting or in the real world of work. Here's where performance-based testing rises to the fore. Requiring students to demonstrate what they have learned and to apply it in a realistic context that closely approximates an on-the-job situation measures how well students can do what the course intended to teach them. As emphasized in *Exceptional Teaching*, "Authentic, performance-based assessments ask students to integrate what they have learned and apply it to resolve an issue, solve a problem, create something new, work collaboratively, or use their written and oral communication skills. Authentic assessments stress the process of learning as well as the outcomes of learning."

Typically, instructors develop an assessment strategy that uses the strengths of both major types of assessments, and the assessment resources developed to support *Pharmacology for Technicians, Fifth Edition* provide ample opportunity for both objective-based and performance-based assessment.

- End-of-chapter work in the textbook provides both objective items and performance-based activities.
- The Test Bank provides objective-based questions for each chapter.
- The Study Partner CD provides objective-based quizzing and matching exercises.

Creating a Grading Plan

By choosing the types of assessments that will measure students' achievement of course and program outcomes, you will already have established a schema of the major grading components. The next step is to weight the scores as preparation for entering them into a grade-calculation system, for example, an Excel spreadsheet.

Will you include non-achievement factors, such as effort and attendance, in students' grades? If so, consider how to measure those elements. While it is simple to track attendance, it is not so easy to objectively evaluate effort and attitude. Some experts recommend that teachers provide regular verbal and written feedback on non-achievement factors, but confine grades to academic achievement.

The following grading plan offers a starting point as you develop your comprehensive grading strategy for a course using *Pharmacology for Technicians, Fifth Edition*:

Attendance	5%
Homework, including Study Partner Reported Mode quizzes	30%
Team reports	10%
Chapter quizzes	10%
Unit tests	25%
Final exam	20%

For More Information

Much of the content of this "Planning the Course" article is based on information found in *Exceptional Teaching: Ideas in Action*. To order a copy of this resource, please visit www.emcp.com or call or e-mail Customer Care at 800-535-6865, educate@emcp.com.

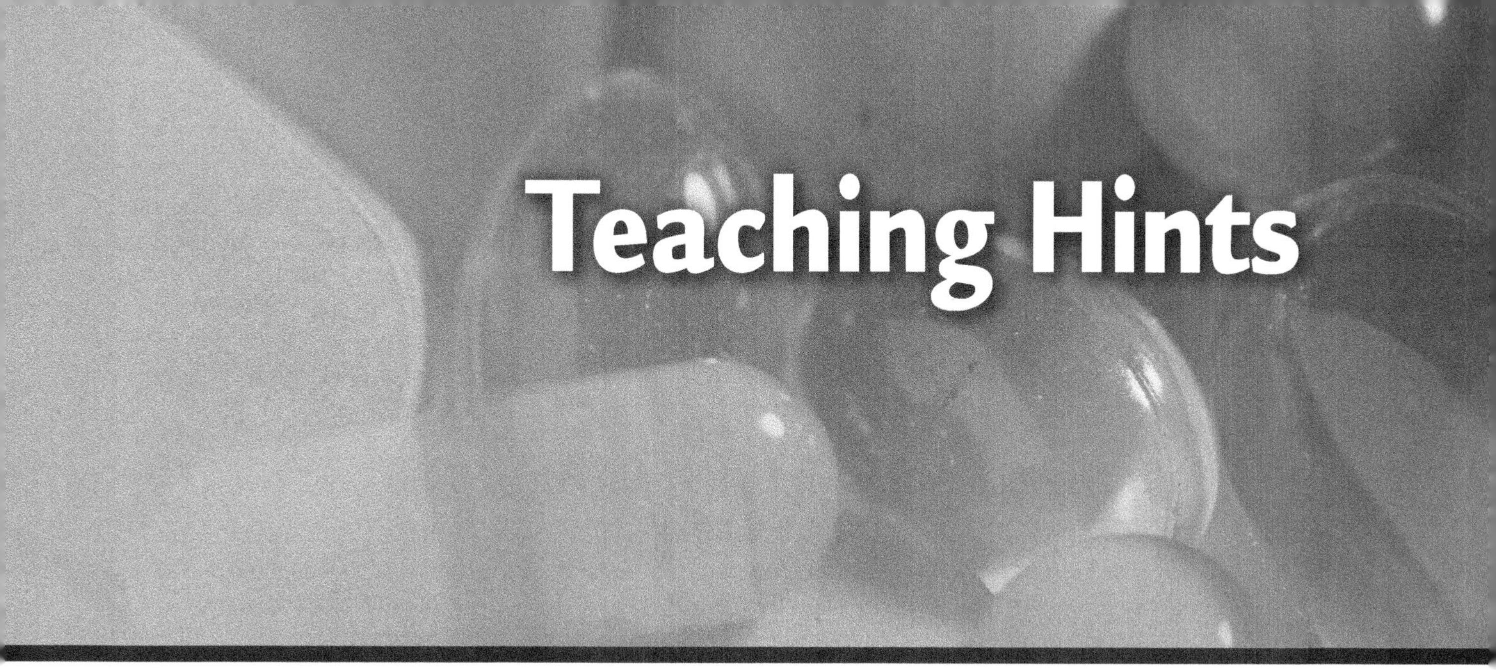

Teaching Hints

Teaching hints help identify key issues discussed in each chapter and provide instructional points to help your students learn chapter content.

Unit 1 Introduction to Pharmacology

Chapter 1 Evolution of Medicinal Drugs

Chapter 1 provides a brief history of pharmacology, explains the role of the pharmacist and pharmacy technician in present-day pharmacology practice, and introduces the student to terminology that will be used frequently in the teaching of drugs. The chapter includes a discussion of the drug legislation and regulation system as well as the process for drug testing and approval.

You may want to create overheads of C-IIs, C-IIIs, and C-IVs and ask the students to identify these substances. Table 1.5 presents these concepts. Narcotics are studied in more detail in Chapter 6. This also might be a good time to compare and contrast the roles of the pharmacist and the pharmacy technician (bullet points on pages 8 and 9) and explain that these roles might vary by state. Students could perhaps be asked to check with their state pharmacy board as to the unique regulations of their state.

Lexi-comp's Drug Information Handbook, Facts and Comparisons, the *Physician's Drug Handbook,* and the FDA website are all good references. You cannot teach students everything there is to know about drugs, but you can equip them with the tools to access the information.

On the first day of class, show the PowerPoint presentation that provides an overview of the study tools available to students in the textbook, Study Partner CD, IRC, and Workbook. This presentation is available on both the student and the instructor sides of the IRC.

Chapter 2 Basic Concepts of Pharmacology

Chapter 2 continues the introduction of concepts and terms that will be used by the pharmacy technician. The mechanisms of drug action (also known as pharmacodynamics) as well as pharmacokinetics are covered. The instructor should stress the four key components of pharmacokinetics—absorption, distribution, metabolism, and elimination (ADME)—as these elements will be addressed continuously throughout the textbook. All drugs have side effects, potentially both beneficial and harmful, and these effects must be considered when a drug is prescribed. This concept should be stressed when teaching this chapter. Additionally, students should be introduced to the concept of drug interactions, because the more drugs a patient takes, the more likely he or she is to encounter a dangerous drug interaction (page 30). Pharmacists and pharmacy technicians must be aware of potential drug interactions when filling and dispensing prescriptions (Chapter 3).

Chapter 3 Dispensing Medications

In Chapter 3, students are introduced to the prescription, the "rights" for correct drug administration, and the dosage forms and routes of administration. The sigs should be memorized, and students should be given prescriptions to work with so that they gain experience working with the real thing. Write out some sample prescriptions in legible handwriting; then give students prescriptions with actual physician handwriting, making sure to observe HIPAA requirements for confidentiality. This also might be a good time to introduce the switch to e-prescribing. Pharmacy technicians should also become familiar with medication labels on dispensing containers, as errors can have fatal consequences.

A good exercise would be to have students create a table of each major route of drug administration (Table 3.3) and list the advantages and disadvantages of each route. It would also be a good idea to go back to this table later in the course and have students give examples of drugs that are administered by each route.

The manner in which the body handles a drug is an important consideration, and this is also discussed. Factors that influence drug action are addressed, especially for elderly and pediatric patients. Endogenous chemicals that affect drug actions and response are also discussed. Because there is increasing controversy in the general public about the relationship between immunizations and autism, this might provide an interesting topic for an open discussion. This is a particularly relevant topic, because there is growing interest in allowing pharmacists to administer certain vaccines. The chapter presents issues related to teaching patients medication management. Instructors may develop specific scenarios to help pharmacy technicians learn which questions they may answer versus those that **must** be answered by a pharmacist.

Unit 2 Major Classes of Pharmaceutical Products I

Chapter 4 Antibiotics

Chapter 4 covers antibiotics as the first drug class. Antobiotics are a good starting point, since most people are familiar with this class of drugs. The concept of bacterial infection is easily understood, as is the idea that antibiotics work by affecting processes unique to bacteria and not present in humans. The difficulty in this topic is the sheer number of drugs and the similarity of their names. This book emphasizes the labels that should accompany each medication and the dispensing techniques that should be used, rather than the clinical aspects of the drugs, as this is beyond the scope of the profession. The clinical information presented helps the technician to make intelligent decisions in dispensing the medication.

Obtain samples of actual warning labels that go on bottles, and let the students determine which ones should be placed on which drugs.

At the end of the chapter, as with all the drug group chapters, a list of the drugs studied is provided. Choose the drugs most familiar to you or most commonly used in your area. Have the students put these drugs on 3 × 5 cards and memorize them. Students can also use the drug flash card tool on the student IRC to create and customize flash cards.

Certain classes of drugs, such as the antibiotics, contain more medications than others. Because of this, these chapters may not go into as much depth about each individual medication, although the most common ones will still be covered in full. Note that, with some drugs, it is more important to identify drug classes than brand and generic names.

It is imperative that each student have a drug handbook and understand how to use it. Many good drug handbooks are available in paper, PDA, or online formats. We cannot possibly teach students everything there is to know about drugs, but we can teach them to locate the information. For example, dosing is highly individual, depending on the patient's condition, the disease state being treated, and so on. It is certainly beyond the scope of this book to provide this information for all cases, but it is important to teach students the key factors they should be aware of to understand proper dosing.

Ceilings are identified, and limited dosing information is provided, but it is in the student's best interest to look up the drugs in standard pharmaceutical references. As pharmacy technicians, they will be doing very little dosing. They will need to be able to recognize errors in dosing, but this will come with experience and is not something that should be memorized.

Pharmacy technicians will frequently be asked by patients or their parents why they were *not* prescribed an antibiotic. This might be a good assignment opportunity for students to create a document explaining that antibiotics are only used for bacterial infections, etc.

Chapter 5 Therapy for Fungal and Viral Infections

Chapter 5 discusses antifungals and antivirals. There are fewer drugs in these categories, but they are being used widely now and are dispensed frequently, often because patients treated with antibiotics may develop opportunistic fungal infections. Because these drugs are so new, few generics are available. The students need to develop a feel for drug classes and how they have similar side effect profiles, but at the same time, the individual differences in the drugs need to be pointed out to the students so that they will better understand the dispensing process and how and why drugs may be used for certain purposes. They also need to develop an understanding of how one drug may be used for more than one disease state. Also emphasize the point that some patients, especially immunocompromised patients, may have to be treated with both antifungals and antivirals. It is also important to stress that, although symptoms that follow infections with viral and bacterial infections may be similar, viral infections do not respond to antibiotics.

In the last decade or so, many antiviral drugs have been developed to treat HIV/AIDS, causing this disease to be seen as a lifelong chronic illness rather than a lethal diagnosis. This is currently the fastest growing area of antiviral drug medications.

Chapter 6 Anesthetics and Narcotics

Chapter 6 describes the central nervous system (CNS) and the peripheral nervous system (PNS) and emphasizes neurotransmitters, the chemicals that underlie the effect of most medications. The pharmacy technician student does not need detailed study of these body systems. However, it is very important that the pharmacy technician be somewhat familiar with neurotransmitters, especially if the technician works in a hospital setting, as many drugs he or she will dispense have both desirable and adverse effects mediated by the nervous system. Less emphasis is placed on anesthesia, and more is placed on narcotics and other analgesics.

The pharmacy technician will frequently face the issue of pain and its appropriate treatment. The pharmacy technician needs to be familiar with these drugs and their classes, including the advantages and disadvantages of the two key classes of analgesic drugs, the narcotic and non-narcotic analgesics. This could be a good time to review DEA schedules and where each narcotic covered in the chapter fits into that schedule.

The instructor will need to emphasize the presence of acetaminophen (Percocet) or its absence (Oxycontin) in the various narcotic-NSAID combinations. It is important for the technician to calculate the acetaminophen content, because high doses of narcotic drug combinations containing acetaminophen can lead to liver damage and possibly death.

Chapter 7 Psychiatric and Related Drugs

In Chapter 7, the emphasis is on identifying drug classes. When students are able to place a drug in a particular category, they will be able to identify adverse reactions, choose the proper warning labels, and be aware of the disease states being treated.

Once a drug's class has been identified, the student should remember a distinguishing characteristic that sets the drug apart within that particular class. This will help the student remember and identify the drug. It may be useful to stress that, unlike the other drugs covered in this chapter, antidepressants do not work rapidly. The delay in clinical improvement may last for weeks. Moreover, older antidepressant medications are highly toxic drugs that may be dispensed (per doctor's orders) in small quantities.

Chapter 8 Drugs for Central Nervous System Disorders

In Chapter 8, the emphasis is still on drug classes. Be sure to point out how a drug can fit into more than one class and how drugs may treat more than one disease state. This is an important concept for the students to understand.

In recent years, as our understanding of the mechanism underlying many neurological disorders has improved, there has been a rapid increase in the number of drugs to treat these disorders. Several of the drugs covered in this chapter were not in clinical use as little as four years ago, and the number is expected to grow rapidly in the next few years.

It is imperative that the pharmacy technician be aware of the narrow therapeutic range of anticonvulsants. It is important to shake phenytoin before giving a dose to a patient. The bottle can be stored upside down to equalize doses. Also, many anticonvulsant drugs are used to treat conditions other than epilepsy. These include certain pain and psychiatric conditions.

The student needs to understand the drugs used for Parkinson's disease and to recognize that, as the disease progresses, the drug effectiveness often diminishes.

It is also important to understand that different classes of drugs are used to treat ADHD/ADD. Many of these medications have abuse potential and are DEA-scheduled drugs.

A large amount of research has been invested in recent years to better understand Alzheimer's disease and its treatment. Several drugs have been released in recent years to treat this disorder, and several more are in the channel.

Multiple sclerosis is a disease requiring very expensive therapy. The technician needs to be aware of the cost of the drugs as well as the storage precautions to be taken when dispensing the drugs. Emphasize the flu-like side effects and the prophylaxis to lessen these symptoms. If time is limited and you need to leave out a section, the one on myasthenia gravis is probably the least important.

Chapter 9 Respiratory Drugs

Chapter 9 begins with the asthma drugs. These are the drugs dispensed most frequently. Young patients, in particular, may have difficulty in properly using inhalers. These patients or their family members should be referred to the pharmacist for consultation. It is important to recognize if a patient is filling a bronchodilator more often than prescribed, as this may indicate a worsening of the underlying disease and may require additional or alternative drug therapy. Several other respiratory disease states (e.g., COPD, emphysema, and chronic bronchitis) are treated with most of these same drugs.

Smoking cessation drugs are important because many of these drugs are now available without a prescription. Pharmacy technicians can use their expertise to help patients with these medications. Be sure to emphasize that the technician should always defer to the pharmacist in areas that require judgment decisions.

Chapter 9 differentiates antitussives, expectorants, decongestants, and antihistamines. The student should be made aware of the different mechanisms of action of each of these drugs. They are easily confused because they are used to treat related symptoms. Moreover, most of the drugs in this class are sold OTC and are taken without doctor's orders. The role of the pharmacist and the pharmacy technician can be vital to the health and well-being of the patient.

The pharmacy technician will frequently be dealing with these drugs, so it is important that the technician have a knowledge of the drugs and drug combinations. The technician should never recommend or discourage the use of a drug; this should be deferred to the pharmacist. However, it is perfectly acceptable for the technician to inform the patient of the contents of the drug.

Unit 3 Major Classes of Pharmaceutical Products II

Chapter 10 Drugs for Gastrointestinal and Related Diseases

Most drugs for treating GI difficulties (indigestion, constipation, diarrhea) are sold OTC and are often taken by patients without a doctor's supervision. Pharmacy technician students should be aware that almost all peptic ulcers are caused by NSAIDs or infection. Thus, it is possible today not just to treat an ulcer, but to cure it.

Diarrhea, while usually not life-threatening, can be fatal if it is prolonged or very severe, as it can cause severe electrolyte disturbances. When feasible, patients asking about such medications should speak directly to the pharmacist.

This chapter emphasizes how these drugs should be administered and their side effects and potential drug interactions. The pharmacy technician cannot recommend drugs or offer counsel regarding these drugs, but he or she should be aware of the names of the most common drugs and the class in which they belong. Flash cards may provide a useful tool to facilitate studying this content. This is also an excellent area in which to incorporate the training of the pharmacy technician. The technician certainly may be called on to explain the difference between an antacid, an H_2 blocker, and a "pump" inhibitor, as well as show the patients where the OTC drugs are stocked.

Obesity is a growing problem in America, and it may be treated with a drug (in addition to changes in diet and behavior). Some drugs may have abuse potential (Dexedrine), while others (Alli) are sold OTC but have potentially unpleasant side effects. The pharmacy technician may be asked questions about these drugs and should be somewhat familiar with them.

Chapter 11 Renal System Drugs

The kidneys are the most important organ system in the body for maintaining water and electrolyte balance. Chapter 11 deals with drugs used to treat assorted renal disorders, including urinary tract infections. UTIs are among the most common infections (particularly in women) to be encountered by the pharmacy technician. Pharmacy technicians should also recognize the quickly increasing number of drugs used to treat benign prostatic hyperplasia in men and the mechanisms by which they work.

The most commonly used drugs acting via the kidneys are the diuretics (hence the reason they are covered in this chapter). Despite their site of action in the kidney, however, they are used for a variety of clinical conditions, particularly cardiac problems. Emphasize the different ways that diuretics work.

Chapter 12 Drugs for Cardiovascular Diseases

There are many cardiovascular conditions, including hypertension, heart failure, and arrhythmias, that may be treated pharmacologically. There are a multitude of cardiovascular drugs, and some (such as Inderal) are used for multiple conditions. This can be very confusing for the student.

Emphasis should be placed on the dispensing of the drugs rather than on their uses. Broad concepts are presented so that the students will better understand each drug and know which label goes on which drug, how often the drug should be taken, and so on.

However, understanding the usage of these drugs and their overlapping uses and conditions will enable the technician to do a better job of dispensing. Each drug needs to be identified by class. It may help for the students to create a chart of the most common cardiac problems and the most common drugs used to treat these conditions.

Emphasis should also be placed on the fact that, for heparin, doses are written in units of activity and not milliliters because heparin is provided by the manufacturer in many different strengths. If a prescription indicates milliliters of heparin, the technician should always verify units with the pharmacist or doctor.

Chapter 13 Drugs for Muscle and Joint Disease and Pain

Although many drugs for joint pain and inflammation are covered in Chapter 13, the most important class, in terms of sheer numbers, are the nonsteroidal anti-inflammatory drugs or NSAIDs. The NSAIDs are a class of drugs that the pharmacy technician will deal with on a daily basis, no matter what the practice setting. Perhaps the single most common complaint of patients visiting a pharmacy is pain, and these are the most common drugs used for that complaint. Students should recognize that, although acetaminophen is often included in this section, it is not truly an NSAID because it is not anti-inflammatory.

This chapter emphasizes the mechanism of action and individual differences in the drugs. Disease states for which these drugs are primarily used are identified. Low-dose aspirin (81 mg) is often used in older patients to reduce the risk of heart attacks and strokes. At one time, this dose of aspirin was used in children and may be referred to as "baby aspirin." However, because of its association with Reye's syndrome, aspirin is no longer used in the pediatric population. Children should be given acetaminophen or ibuprofen.

Chapter 14 Hormonal Disorders and Their Treatment

The endocrine system is one of the two primary systems in the body for communication of information, the other being the nervous system. In the discussion of hormonal systems, the major emphasis is on birth control pills and hormone replacement therapy, both for females, because these groups of medications are among the most frequently dispensed. Today, however, many males are prescribed drugs for erectile dysfunction, some of which may have potentially life-threatening adverse effects.

Other topics included in Chapter 14 are drugs used to correct thyroid hormone imbalance and thyroid dysfunction, adrenal sex hormones, drugs to treat osteoporosis, bacterial STDs, corticosteroids for inflammation, and hypoglycemic agents for diabetes.

Prescriptions for thyroid medications are usually "Dispense as Written," to maintain consistent blood levels of drug. Pharmacy computer programs often will automatically switch to the generic equivalent. The pharmacy technician may need to switch the drug back to the brand name. This can be used as a teaching opportunity for the student.

Students should recognize the similarities and differences between type 1 and type 2 diabetes and which drugs are appropriate for each type. Students should understand that injectable insulin is available in several forms that differ in duration of action and are not interchangeable. A patient is commonly prescribed multiple forms of insulin to be taken throughout the day. Also, patients with type 2 diabetes can be treated with oral hypoglycemic agents or injectable insulin, whereas only insulin can be used for type 1 diabetes.

Chapter 15 Topical, Ophthalmic, and Otic Medications

Drugs discussed in Chapter 15 range from chemicals used to diminish acne to those used to treat skin cancer. Drugs used to treat both eye and ear ailments are also covered.

Pharmacy technician students should recognize the most common skin conditions and be familiar with prototype drugs to treat these conditions. Students may use Internet resources to help identify the most common drugs used for each of the categories in the tables within this chapter. Treating skin problems requires many medications in many forms. Several topical medications are OTC drugs, which presents the pharmacy technician with an opportunity to provide information to consumers.

Isotrentoin provides a teaching opportunity because it requires a complex series of steps be taken before it can be administered. Ask students why this is, and whether there are other drugs discussed in the course for which such a plan might also be useful.

Students should be able to identify the most common ear and eye ailments and be able to identify prototype drugs as well as identify at-risk populations (e.g., geriatric patients, glaucoma and pediatrics patients, and patients with ear infections).

Unit 4 Chemotherapy and Miscellaneous Pharmaceutical Products

Chapter 16 Recombinant Drugs and Chemotherapy

Chapter 16 deals with the new but rapidly growing area of recombinant DNA drugs. These drugs are created using a process that uses microorganisms to manufacture large quantities of proteins identical to those normally produced in humans. Some view this area as the future of pharmacotherapy. This field is still in its infancy, and only a few drugs are produced in this manner. However, although they are increasing in usage, they are extremely expensive. They are dispensed for hospital use, home infusion, retail, and long-term care. They are very expensive for small operations and hospitals with restricted formularies. It is difficult to carry them in inventory. This is one of the reasons companies are being formed to dispense only these drugs.

The immune system is increasingly becoming a target for drug action. Certain drugs are developed to interfere with the immune system to prevent it from rejecting transplanted organs. Other drugs, monoclonal antibodies, have been developed to enhance the body's own immune system to, for example, fight cancer.

Because chemo drugs are often used in malignant disease states, they are also discussed in this chapter. It is important to know how and when these drugs are used in conjunction with these malignant states and each other.

Chapter 17 Vitamins, OTC Supplements, Antidotes, and Miscellaneous Topics

Chapter 17 discusses substances other than what most consider drugs.

When vitamins are given in quantities higher than those obtained from a normal diet, they may be considered to be drugs. Also, certain foods may be considered "medical food" if they meet strict criteria set by the Food and Drug Administration (FDA).

Pharmacy technicians may be involved in the preparation of enteral nutrition when patients cannot consume food by mouth. For some patients, drugs must be given by vein. In a home infusion company or a hospital, the technician may need to mix total parenteral nutrition on a regular basis, so it is necessary to be aware of the complexities of this process. Although PN is probably the more correct term, TPN (Total Parenteral Nutrition) is more commonly used.

Another area of pharmacy, and one in which the technician will be very much involved, is the growing use of herbals. These medicinal products are becoming more popular, especially in the United States. People are turning to nature as a healing source. These are OTC drugs, so the technician can serve as a resource. A potential issue with these drugs is the minimal oversight by federal regulatory agencies, such aş the FDA, so there is little if any reliable data on the efficacy and safety of these herbals.

Emergency medications are a major responsibility of pharmacy technicians now, because they prepare and keep the carts up to date.

The book ends by focusing on the role that pharmacy technicians will play if this country ever experiences a bioterrorist attack.

End-of-Chapter Questions: Chapter Review

Unit 1 Introduction to Pharmacology

Chapter 1 Evolution of Medicinal Drugs

Understanding Pharmacology

Multiple Choice

1. b
2. b
3. a
4. a
5. b
6. d
7. a
8. c
9. c
10. d

True/False

1. false (Lister introduced antiseptics)
2. false (Hippocrates first performed dissections)
3. true
4. false (Dioscorides wrote this text)
5. true
6. true
7. false (Medication guides and black box warnings are separate things entirely.)
8. true
9. true
10. false (AAPT is run by volunteer pharmacy technicians to promote safe and efficacious dispensing and use of medications.)

Pharmacology at Work

1. Schedule II: cannot be prescribed by phone; no refills; morphine, oxycodone, meperidine, hydromorphone, fentanyl

   Schedule III: can be refilled up to five times in six months if authorized by a physician; codeine with aspirin, codeine with acetaminophen, anabolic steroids
2. Phase I: small number of healthy volunteers

   Phase II: short-term placebo-to-drug comparisons

   Phase III: placebo-to-drug, dose escalation

   Phase IV: long-term safety and efficacy

   Eliminating the fourth step would eliminate safety. Also, the drug companies would not know whether they could make a profit. This might affect whether or not they manufacture the drug on a larger scale.
3. a. same batch requirements
   b. identical in strength, dosage form, and route of administration
   c. same use indications
   d. same batch requirements for identity, strength, dosage form, and route of administration

e. must yield similar blood absorption and urinary excretion curves for the active ingredient.

Some might prefer generics to save money. Others may believe that generic drugs are not as good as brand-name drugs.

Internet Research

1. National certification is highly desirable for potential employees. Other qualities such as strong communication skills, knowledge of medication names, and an understanding of medical terminology are also desirable. This course will help students succeed in the job market by enabling them to demonstrate knowledge of the field during the interview process and providing them with an educational background that demonstrates their commitment to the field. Internet sources include the U.S. Department of Labor's Bureau of Labor Statistics (www.stats.bls.gov) and the Pharmacy Technician Certification Board (www.ptcb.org).
2. The object of this exercise is for the student to become familiar with the overall scope of the FDA and to become acquainted with its website as a valuable source of information. Student responses will vary depending on the topic researched but should include some critical thinking related to the impact of the regulatory process on the marketing of drugs. The FDA's website is www.fda.gov.

Reflecting on the Profession

1. Students may discuss customer service, chemistry lab experience, or retail experience. Part-time work, especially in a pharmacy, could be quite helpful.
2. Students could do online research or interview a pharmacy technician or pharmacist. They may have other ideas as well.

Chapter 2 Basic Concepts of Pharmacology

Understanding Pharmacology

Multiple Choice

1. a
2. c
3. c
4. a
5. b
6. d
7. c
8. b
9. a
10. d

True/False

1. true
2. false, addition
3. false, potentiation
4. false, 50%
5. false, it does affect absorption
6. true
7. true
8. true
9. false, most drugs cannot pass through
10. true

Pharmacology at Work

1. Different drugs have different effects on individuals. The effects of the body's chemicals must be considered as well as the effects the drug has on the body. Each person's body will have a different rate of absorption, distribution, metabolism, and excretion depending on many factors.
2. Receptor: A group of specific protein molecules with which drugs combine reversibly or irreversibly. The basic requirement for a receptor is the ability to discriminate a signal.

   Agonist: A drug that binds to a receptor to elicit the natural biological response.

   Antagonist: A drug that interacts with a receptor to prevent biological responses. (For example, an H_2 blocker such as cimetidine blocks the body's response.)
3. Half-life ($T_{1/2}$) is the time necessary for the body to eliminate half of the drug in circulation at any given time. If a drug's half-life is six hours, it would take thirty to forty hours to remove it from the body.
4. Ceiling effect is the point at which the body no longer gets increased response with increased dosing. Further increase will produce no greater therapeutic effect but could actually be detrimental.

Internet Research

1. Through this exercise the student will become acquainted with the National Library of Medicine's PubMed website (www.nlm.nih.gov), an important tool for searching the medical literature, and will see how the concepts covered in the chapter are used in real-world examples. The student should be able to find good examples simply by searching on the keyword "pharmacokinetic." If the students are struggling to find abstracts that use the terms introduced in the chapter, you may want to direct them to focus on articles that use the term "pharmacokinetic" within the title. Article citations should include the article title, author(s), journal name, date of publication, and page numbers.
2. Many Internet sites will discuss the issue of grapefruit juice interactions. Review the sources to confirm that the sites provided by the students are credible sites. Also, compare the different lists and discuss why there might be inconsistencies.

Reflecting on the Profession

1. Students may discuss flash cards and practice quizzes (both of which are available on the Student CD), as well as sketching body systems and small-group review. Encourage them to share ideas.
2. Students' answers will vary. Regardless of position, students should support their opinions and demonstrate critical thinking on the topic.

Chapter 3 Dispensing Medications

Understanding Pharmacology

Multiple Choice

1. d
2. d
3. a
4. d
5. b
6. b
7. d
8. b
9. d
10. a

True/False

1. false, all controlled substances must have the prescriber's DEA number on the prescription
2. true
3. false, it must be handwritten in most states
4. false, the elderly spend a lot of money on drugs; it is a big concern
5. false, constipation is a problem
6. false, age and weight and disease state must be considered
7. false, body surface is best, but weight is most often used
8. true
9. true
10. false, the ear only

Matching

1. a
2. c
3. d
4. b
5. g
6. e
7. h
8. f
9. j
10. i
11. k
12. l
13. m
14. p
15. o
16. n
17. t
18. s
19. r
20. q

Pharmacology at Work

1. The patient's name and the date the prescription was written.

   The inscription, which states the name, dose, and quantities of the ingredients.

The signa, which gives directions to be included on the label for the patient to follow in taking the medication.

An indication of the number of refills allowed, or "no refills" if that is the case.

The signature and address of the prescribing physician.

Indication of whether generic substitution is permitted.

2. Patient name, date the prescription was filled, inscription, signa and number of refills, physician's name, prescription number, pharmacy address, and expiration date.
3. Absorption, distribution, clearance, metabolism, and excretion all change with age.
4. Reevaluate all dosages at regular intervals. Be sure the dosage is appropriate for the child's weight/age. Always double-check all computations.

Internet Research

1. According to http://www.cdc.gov/flu/protect/vaccine.htm, those at high risk such as healthcare workers, all children aged 6 months to 23 months, adults aged 65 years or older, and pregnant women in their second or third trimester should get the flu vaccine during the influenza season. Students might also find http://www.cdc.gov/flu/keyfacts.htm helpful in researching this question.
2. Because of the potential for misreading abbreviations, many abbreviations that had been commonly used are now considered dangerous. The ISMP provides a list of dangerous abbreviations and keeps this list up-to-date at its website, http://www.ismp.org. Some states have taken steps to further diminish the potential for tampering with medication orders as well as for misreading them by requiring that medication orders be printed or typewritten, and numbers be written out.

Reflecting on the Profession

1. Students will likely discuss patient safety, privacy, differing levels of training and education, and the law. A student who doesn't like the policy on patient counseling must recognize the law, but may provide interesting support for this position.
2. Encourage students to share interesting resources with one another.

Unit 2 Major Classes of Pharmaceutical Products I

Chapter 4 Antibiotics

Pharmaceuticals and Body Functions

Multiple Choice

1. a
2. d
3. b
4. c
5. d
6. d
7. b
8. b
9. b
10. a

True/False

1. false; nausea, vomiting, flushing, increased blood pressure
2. false, cannot
3. true
4. false, PCN
5. false, 1% chance
6. false, hospital
7. false, not
8. true (unrelative colitis = GI upset)
9. true
10. true

Diseases and Drug Therapies

1. Preventing folic acid synthesis, inhibiting cell wall formation, blocking protein formation, interfering with nucleic acid formation, disrupting cell membranes, and disrupting nucleic acid structure.
2. Three of the following:
   Augmentin: amoxicillin-clavulanate
   Unasyn: ampicillin-sulbactam
   Timentin: ticarcillin-clavulanate
   Zosyn: piperacillin-tazobactam
3. Urinary tract, otitis media, ulcerative colitis, lower respiratory, general.
4. Bactericidal: kills bacteria.
   Bacteriostatic: inhibits growth of bacteria.
5. Nosocomial: hospital acquired.
   Community: acquired outside of hospital setting.
6. Superinfection: a new infection complicating the course of therapy of an existing infection, due to invasion by bacteria or fungi resistant to the drugs in use.
7. Avoid the sun. Drink lots of water. Finish all medication. Take on an empty stomach.
   The first two are the most important; the others could be put on almost any antibiotic.
8. Penicillin binds to penicillin-binding proteins of the bacteria and interferes with synthesis of the cell wall.
9. Because it contains a lot of sugar.
10. Patient and partner should be treated and both should refrain from sex for several days.
11. First dose is larger than successive doses.
12. Particles of sulfa will be on the tray and could stick to the next drug you place on the tray. If someone is allergic to sulfa—and quite a few people are—then that patient would have an allergic reaction to sulfa and think they are allergic to another drug.
13. Not to drink alcohol.
14. Unnecessary prescribing and patient noncompliance.
15. Empirical treatment is using a broad-spectrum antibiotic on an unidentified infection.
    It is often used in order to begin therapy immediately when there is not enough time to wait for lab tests to come back identifying the causative organism of the infection.

Dispensing Medications

1. Cleocin or Zithromax
2. Take four capsules prior to procedure. Dispense four capsules.
3. Take two immediately, then one each day (days 2–5) until finished. Dispense six capsules, 250 mg.
4. Student should create a chart that contains the following information:

Tetracyclines

demeclocycline (Declomycin)
doxycycline (Vibramycin)
minocycline (Minocin)
tetracycline (Sumycin)

Quinolones

ciprofloxacin (Ciloxan, Cipro)
gatifloxacin (Tequin)
gemifloxacin (Factive)
levofloxacin (Levaquin)
moxifloxacin (Avelox, Vigamox)
norfloxacin (Noroxin)
ofloxacin (Floxin, Ocuflox)

Sulfonamides

sulfamethoxazole-trimethoprim (Bactrim DS, Septra DS)
sulfasalazine (Azulfidine)
sulfisoxazole (Gantrisin)

Cephalosporins

ceftriaxone (Rocephin)
cefazolin (Ancef)

Others

nitrofurantoin (Macrobid, Macrodantin)
azithromycin (Zithromax)

Internet Research

1. The student's report should note that (1) the overuse of antibiotics endangers their effectiveness, and (2) there are ongoing efforts to curb the use of antibiotics. This exercise requires the student to think critically about how the presentation of information, which varies among different media sources, affects the reader's understanding of a particular topic. While the student may or may not find differences

of opinion, most will observe a difference of emphasis among the sites. The World Health Organization (WHO) at http://www.who.int and the Centers for Disease Control (CDC) at http://www.cdc.gov cover this topic. Popular press sources will range from *Scientific American* to CNN and ABC.

2. Many of the disease states mentioned in this chapter will have entire websites devoted to their discussion. This exercise introduces the student to critical disease state concepts such as etiology and will help the student to view drug therapy within the larger context of diagnosis, evaluation, and treatment.

Reflecting on the Profession

1. Encourage students to share their experiences.
2. Students may discuss flash cards and practice quizzes (both of which are available on the Study Guide CD) as well as small-group review. Encourage them to share ideas.

What Would You Do?

1. The technician may tell the mother that the drug must be kept in the refrigerator, but cannot recommend a dosing schedule.
2. No. Discussing that kind of information would need to be handled by the pharmacist.

Chapter 5 Therapy for Fungal and Viral Infections

Pharmaceuticals and Body Functions

Multiple Choice

1. c
2. b
3. c
4. a
5. b
6. a
7. a
8. a
9. b
10. d

True/False

1. true
2. false, with a fatty meal and avoid the sun
3. true
4. true
5. true
6. false, a virus can
7. false, they are at risk
8. false, not suppository
9. true
10. true

Diseases and Drug Therapies

1. Acute, chronic, slow; or by targeted area: local, general
2. To avoid precipitation
3. Dose one week per month
4. Nausea, anorexia, vomiting
5. Some viruses can lie dormant and then under certain conditions reproduce and behave like infective agents.

Dispensing Medications

1. a. 68.18 mg
   b. amount of D_5W missing; no premeds ordered
2. a. 4.9 g
   b. hydration
3. a. lamivudine #56, zidovudine #56
   b. PEP needle stick or exposure

Internet Research

1. AIDS drugs are emerging rapidly, and this exercise functions as an addendum to the text, ensuring that the student becomes familiar with some of the newer drugs. The FDA indexes product release announcements for new AIDS drugs and will be a good source of information for this exercise. AIDS portal sites, such as AIDSmeds.com (www.aidsmeds.com), also provide links to this type of information.
2. The spread of viral diseases such as AIDS is carefully tracked by public health organizations on the national and international level. This exercise introduces the student to the concept of tracking disease state populations and to the main sources of these population data: WHO (www.who.

int) and the CDC (www.cdc.gov). Each of these organizations details its methodology in terms of how it collects its data and notes the limitations of its methods. The student might observe that this process is quite complex and involves a good deal of data extrapolation. You may want to lead a class discussion about the importance of tracking this type of information, especially in the instance of AIDS. Point out that public health organizations need to understand the prevalence of the disease state in order to allocate research and healthcare funds and to target public outreach and education programs appropriately. You may choose to direct students to www.aidsinfo.org.

Reflecting on the Profession

1. Students will likely discuss maintaining a clean and sterile work environment, frequent hand washing, wearing gloves and mask when appropriate, avoiding needle pricks, and professional behavior.
2. Students may discuss flash cards and practice quizzes (both of which are available on the Study Guide CD) as well as small-group review and online research. Encourage them to share ideas.

What Would You Do?

1. Unlike other drug classes, the HIV drugs are used for only one disease. HIV cannot be transmitted through normal contact with the patient. Contagion may actually be a concern if the patient has the flu or TB, because these diseases can be transmitted through airborne particles, but HIV is transmitted only through contact with body fluids. Technicians, like other healthcare workers, must of course be in the habit of frequent hand washing. This will help prevent flu during the flu season. Technicians also must wipe down the counters and phones with alcohol on a regular basis, no matter what the setting. The telephone is a great source to communicate diseases. The AIDS patient, however, deserves the same respect as any other patient. No one should be judged by his or her disease.
2. Get a cleaner like Clorox from the cleaning supplies; HIV is a relatively weak virus, and Clorox will kill it on surfaces.

Chapter 6 Anesthetics and Narcotics

Pharmaceuticals and Body Functions

Multiple Choice

1. b
2. d
3. c
4. a
5. c
6. d
7. b
8. b
9. a
10. e

True/False

1. true
2. true
3. true
4. true
5. false, vasoconstriction
6. true
7. true
8. false, small unmyelinated first and larger myelinated last
9. true
10. true

Matching

1. a
2. d
3. a
4. c
5. d
6. a
7. a
8. d
9. d
10. b
11. b
12. b
13. d
14. c
15. a

16. d
17. d
18. b
19. d
20. a
21. a
22. a
23. a
24. d
25. a
26. d
27. b
28. a

Diseases and Drug Therapies

1. a. goals: amnesia, adequate muscle relaxation, adequate ventilation, pain control
   b. indices: blood pressure, pulse, urinary output, oxygen, respiration, tissue perfusion, hypovolemia/hypervolemia
2. a. advantages: all types of nerve tissue are affected, reversible, no residual damage
   b. pain perception, temperature, touch sensation, proprioception, skeletal muscle tone
3. a. classification: acute, chronic, malignant
   b. major sources: somatic (bones, muscles, ligaments); visceral (kidneys, intestines, liver); neuropathic (nerves); sympathetic (overactivity in sympathetic system)
4. a. analgesia, sedation, euphoria and dysphoria, cough reflex
   b. analgesic ladder: NSAIDs; NSAIDs plus "weak" opioid; strong opioid with adjuvant analgesic

Dispensing Medications

1. Simple analgesics: aspirin, acetaminophen
   NSAIDs
   Ergotamine or Midrin
   Imitrex
   Stadol
   Reglan for nausea
   Triptans are considered the drug of choice for treatment of migraine management.
   Inderal is the drug of choice for prophylaxis.
   (Remember, migraines are very patient-specific; therefore, these are not the only correct answers. Due to side effect profile, and so on, these are the most common choices. Also, with the new drugs on the market, ergotamine is being used less and less.)
2. In case a patient develops malignant hyperthermia
3. a. nitrous oxide
   b. fentanyl

Internet Research

1. Some of the drugs covered in this chapter fall under the confines of the Controlled Substances Act (CSA). This exercise enables the student to reexamine this important legislation (which was introduced in Chapter 1) through a survey of current, real-world issues. A substantial amount of state and national legislative news is indexed online. Popular press sources such as CNN and *USA Today* may also cover stories related to new CSA legislation.
2. Through this exercise, students will recognize that the thinking relative to the appropriate use of pharmaceuticals continues to evolve. Standards and guidelines ensure that patients receive proper and consistent care. These guidelines also help physicians make good judgments with regard to the administration of drug therapies. Medscape (www.medscape.com) has a very comprehensive pain management resource center, and the Federation of State Medical Boards of the United States (www.fsmb.org) also indexes information on the treatment of pain.

Reflecting on the Profession

1. Empathy means understanding and seeing one's self in the situation of another. But too much empathy can hinder professionalism. Encourage students to explore their feelings on this subject.
2. If class time allows, invite a pharmacy technician to speak to your students.

What Would You Do?

1. The patient has obviously altered the prescription. The first thing to do would be to call the MD, and make sure the prescription was not for #80. After that, it is truly up to the policies of the pharmacy, the MD, and

the pharmacist. The important thing for the technician would be to show appropriate empathy for the patient in this situation.

2. You cannot sell only the controlled substance. It is legal to do so, but not ethical. The antibiotic is going to make the patient well, while the narcotic is only going to mask the symptoms. You can sell the antibiotic without the narcotic. If patient does not understand, get the pharmacist. In fact, this is actually a pharmacist's decision. If the pharmacist tells you to sell the narcotic without the antibiotic, you are not breaking the law.

Chapter 7 Psychiatric and Related Drugs

Pharmaceuticals and Body Functions

Multiple Choice

1. c
2. a
3. d
4. d
5. b
6. d
7. c
8. d
9. d
10. d

True/False

1. false, benzodiazepines
2. false, there are others
3. true
4. true
5. true
6. true
7. true
8. false, they have abuse potential, and now the Z hypnotics are first-line
9. true
10. false, good choice in elderly, but poor choice in young

Diseases and Drug Therapies

1. Five of the following: pessimism, worry, intense sadness, loss of concentration, slowing of mental processes, problems eating and/or sleeping, a feeling that life has no meaning.
2. Five of the following: elevated or irritable mood; increase in activity (socially, at work, sexually); pressure to keep talking; racing thoughts; grandiose ideas; decreased need for sleep; distractibility; excessive involvement in activities with a high potential for painful consequences, such as buying sprees, sexual indiscretions, foolish business investments, or reckless driving; sadness; excessive crying; low energy; loss of pleasure; difficulty concentrating; irritability; thoughts of death or suicide.
3. Four of the following: propranolol, hydroxyzine, BuSpar, amoxapine, trifluoperazine.
4. Alprazolam, (Xanax) lorazepam (Ativan), and oxazepam (Serax).
5. Flurazepam (Dalmane), temazepam (Restoril), triazolam (Halcion), estazolam (ProSom), and quazepam (Doral).
6. Acknowledge problem; limit time spent with substance users; seek professional help; seek support from recovering alcoholics.
7. Nausea, face becoming hot and scarlet, intense throbbing in head and neck, severe headache, difficulty breathing, thirst, chest pain, severe vomiting, uneasiness, confusion, blurred vision.
8. Normalize sleep schedule; increase physical exercise; discontinue alcohol as sedative; sleep only seven to eight hours in a 24-hour period; limit caffeine intake; eliminate any drug that could lead to insomnia.
9. Anticholinergic, cardiovascular, dermatologic, endocrine, hematologic, neurologic, ophthalmologic, withdrawal, sedation, hypotension.
10. Any three of the following: manic, bipolar, unipolar, SAD, PTSD.

Dispensing Medications

For safety reasons, if not state law, all numbers should be written out to avoid possible errors or falsification of amounts. This correction should be noted on all three prescriptions.

1. Only six fillings are allowed (original plus five refills).

2. 1,200 mg/day is too much; 800 mg/day maximum.
3. Duration of therapy should be limited to seven to 10 days; too many refills.

Internet Research

1. The student will need to think critically in order to extract the designated information from among the mass of information most manufacturers provide. Clearly, it is in the best interest of the manufacturer to ensure the accuracy and reliability of any information it publishes on its drugs. In fact, misinformation is prohibited by law. Thus, information obtained through the drug manufacturer's site should be highly reliable. This conclusion may be contrary to the student's first assumption.
2. The student will practice researching disease states and develop an understanding for the role of drug therapy within the larger context of diagnosis, evaluation, and treatment. Some common signs of bipolar disease include irritability, difficulty sleeping, trouble concentrating, excessive energy, and irresponsible behavior. Good Internet sources of information on bipolar mood disorder include the American Academy of Family Physicians (www.aafp.org), Depression and Bipolar Support Alliance (www.dbsalliance.org), and Psycom (psycom.net).

Reflecting on the Profession

1. This is a good opportunity to underscore students' understanding of empathy, nonjudgmental behavior, and professionalism.
2. Encourage students to think about prior experience in retail sales, customer service, lab settings, and more. Direct them to the electronic resources available with the course to begin to work on their resumes.

What Would You Do?

1. The best thing would be to ignore the person as much as possible and concentrate on filling the prescription correctly, but call someone such as security to remove the intoxicated person if he or she becomes abusive. Do not get involved in a discussion, because it is impossible to reason with someone who is inebriated. Inebriation can bring out this abusive nature in some people.
2. No, this is an area where you must be very careful. Mr. Williams is protected by HIPAA; only he can get a printout of his drugs.

Chapter 8 Drugs for Central Nervous System Disorders

Pharmaceuticals and Body Functions

Multiple Choice

1. d
2. a
3. c
4. d
5. c
6. a
7. d
8. b
9. a
10. a

True/False

1. false, Valium
2. false, does not cross
3. false, levodopa (Dopar)
4. false, levodopa-carbidopa (Sinemet)
5. true
6. true
7. true
8. false (must NOT be frozen)
9. true
10. true

Diseases and Drug Therapies

1. Five of the following: epilepsy, genetic causes, congenital causes, trauma, infection, alcohol or drug withdrawal, CV disease, metabolic abnormalities, hyponatremia, hyperglycemia, hypocalcemia, hypoxia, uremia, toxic substances.
2. Resting, firing, return to resting.
3. It does not affect phenobarbital, phenytoin, or primidone.

4. For Parkinson's disease and to dry up milk in nursing mothers.

Dispensing Medications

1. Drying up milk
2. Absence seizures
3. Parkinson's disease
4. Parkinson's disease
5. Flu
6. Parkinson's disease, multiple sclerosis
7. Narcolepsy
8. ADHD/ADD
9. ALS
10. MS

Internet Research

1. This exercise reinforces the concept of clinical trials, which was introduced in Chapter 1, and helps to illustrate the different types of methods and conclusions that correspond to each of the three phases. The National Library of Medicine indexes trials that are currently recruiting patients on its clinical trials site (www.clinicaltrials.gov) and lists the location, phase, and drug being tested.
2. This exercise asks the student to evaluate the quality and utility of information provided by various websites for a particular audience, the patient. The student may observe that some sites are more oriented toward the medical professional and do not provide enough background or practical information for the patient. They may also observe that certain sites are easier to navigate than others and that certain sites have more comprehensive coverage, catering to patients who know very little about their disease and only want practical tips, as well as those who seek a greater depth of understanding.

Reflecting on the Profession

1. Students may discuss flash cards and practice quizzes (both of which are available on the Study Guide CD) as well as sketching the central nervous system and small-group review. Encourage them to share ideas.
2. This is an opportunity for students to personalize the work of the pharmacy technician and strengthen their balance of empathy and professionalism. They might consider volunteering in a clinic or senior facility.

What Would You Do?

1. Because Lyrica is a controlled substance, it cannot have 12 refills. Many prescribers forget that it is a controlled substance. You would need to call the prescriber and explain that a prescription for this drug can only be written for six months.
2. The prescription cannot be filled until the date the doctor has specified.

Chapter 9 Respiratory Drugs

Pharmaceuticals and Body Functions

Multiple Choice

1. a
2. b
3. a
4. b
5. d
6. c
7. b
8. a
9. a
10. c

True/False

1. true
2. true, epi is used for life threatening, not acute
3. false, Serevent is a maintenance drug
4. false, can be
5. false, only asthma
6. false, GI too
7. true
8. true
9. true
10. false, not for birth control

Diseases and Drug Therapies

1. Just be sure the following steps are listed. Hopefully some creativity will emerge using pictures, drawings, etc.

Steps for using a metered dose inhaler (MDI):

1) Remove cap and shake inhaler.
2) Breathe out all the way.
3) Place mouthpiece between lips.
4) Press down on inhaler, hold for a few seconds, breathe in slowly.
5) Hold breath and count to ten.
6) Breathe out slowly.

Steps for using a dry-powder MDI:

1) Activate the inhaler, insert disk, etc.
2) Breathe out all the way.
3) Put the mouthpiece to your lips and breathe in quickly.
4) Hold breath and count to ten.
5) Breathe out slowly.

2. Sleep well every night; be able to go to work or school every day; be free from wheezing all day; have good control of coughing; be able to continue with activities and exercise; tolerate medicines well.
3. Methylxanthines, corticosteroids, beta agonists, and ipratropium bromide.
4. Antihistamine: dries up secretions; decongestant: enables sinus cavity to drain; expectorant: decreases mucus viscosity enabling patients to cough it out more easily; antitussive: suppresses coughing.
5. Clemastine (Tavist).
6. Posters should exemplify some of the side effects of smoking as well as benefits of smoking cessation. Insurance companies are charging higher fees for smokers because they use more drugs and have more illnesses. Public facilities have become "no smoking" areas because of the health benefits. This could turn into a community service project. Things to make sure they include in the posters: improved performance in sports and sex; better-smelling home, car, clothing, and breath; economic savings; freedom from addiction; healthier babies; improved health; improved self-esteem; improved sense of taste and smell; no concern about exposing others to smoke; setting a good example for children and young adults.

Dispensing Medications

1. Set a date.

   Inform family, friends, and coworkers of the decision, and request understanding and support.

   Remove cigarettes from the environment, and avoid spending a lot of time in places where smoking is prevalent.

   Review previous quit attempts, if applicable, and analyze factors associated with relapse.

   Anticipate challenges to the quit attempt, particularly during the critical first few weeks.
2. Serevent is a maintenance drug and should never be used prn. "Use as directed" is unclear. It depends on what is being treated.

   For the maintenance and prevention of asthma: 42 mcg (2 puffs) twice daily (12 hours apart).

   For exercise-induced asthma: 42 mcg (2 puffs) 30–60 minutes prior to exercise. Additional doses should not be used for 12 hours.

   For COPD: 42 mcg (2 puffs) twice daily (12 hours apart). Do not use a spacer with the inhalation powder.
3. 2 mL

   Note: The label printed on page 277 of the textbook is incorrect. Please use this one in its place.

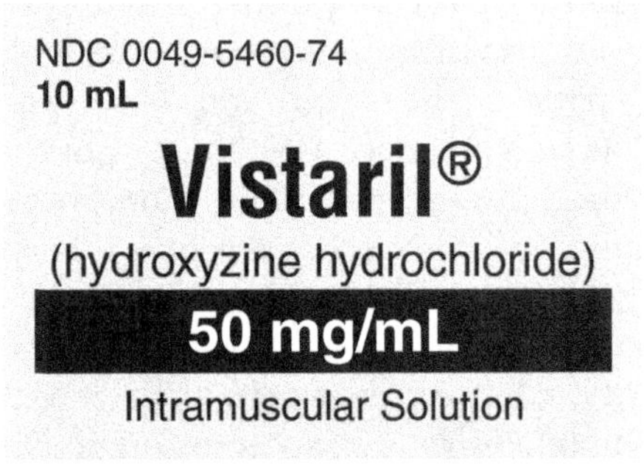

4. Diphenhydramine: drowsiness.
5. Before exposure, because they work better at preventing than treating.

Internet Research

1. Incidence, prevalence, and risk populations are important concepts in the medical profession. This exercise illustrates these concepts through a real-world example. Both WHO (www.who.int) and CDC (www.cdc.gov) index TB statistics.
2. The student will note that many manufacturers dedicate entire websites to a

single prescription medication. For example, Schering-Plough has a site dedicated to Claritin (www.claritin.com). These sites will typically index a significant amount of product information including side effects, FAQs, as well as general information. This exercise requires the student to think critically about the marketing of different types of drugs. During class discussion, you may want to direct the students to the Chapter 1 discussions on the regulatory and drug development processes and ask them whether they think that these processes have any bearing on the way drug companies allocate their marketing resources.

Reflecting on the Profession

1. Students may discuss flash cards and practice quizzes (both of which are available on the Study Guide CD) as well as sketching the pulmonary system and small-group review. Encourage them to share ideas.
2. This is an opportunity for students to think broadly on the layout of a typical pharmacy and where OTC medications can best be shelved. Encourage students to consider ease of access, safety and security, and other factors.

What Would You Do?

1. Normally the technician would follow the pharmacist's instructions. However, there are circumstances where they must not, and one is if the pharmacist is telling them to break the law. Then they must follow the rules and regulations set forth by the government, or they could be held accountable. On this professional decision, one should err on the side of the manufacturer. Nothing bad could happen by putting the date on the box, but if the date is left off and the patient continues to use an expired drug, there could be repercussions.
2. This needs to be handled by the pharmacist. Hopefully, the technician would be encouraged to enroll in a "stop smoking" program.

Unit 3 Major Classes of Pharmaceutical Products II

Chapter 10 Drugs for Gastrointestinal and Related Diseases

Pharmaceuticals and Body Functions

Multiple Choice

1. d
2. b
3. c
4. b
5. a
6. d
7. d
8. b
9. d
10. d

True/False

1. false, Rowasa is an enema; Imuran is an immunosuppressive agent
2. false, Actigall dissolves gallstones
3. false, distension, excessive gas, flatulence
4. false, 80%
5. true
6. false, loperamide is OTC, Lomotil is narcotic
7. false, hepatitis C cannot
8. false, 2 to 3 times ideal body weight
9. true
10. true

Diseases and Drug Therapies

1. Weight loss, plateau, cessation of dieting, resumption of regular eating habits, increase in weight.
2. They provide a sense of fullness because of the fiber, and therefore patients eat less, which results in fewer calories.

3.

Hepatitis A	Hepatitis B	Hepatitis C
Immune globulin (Gamunex)	adefovir (Hepsera)	interferon alfa-2b (Intron A)
	entecavir (Baraclude)	peginterferon alfa-2a (Pegasys)
	interferon alfa-2a (roferon A)	ribavirin (Copegus, Rebetol)
	lamivudine (Epivir, Epivir-HBV)	
	peginterferon alfa-2a (Pegasys)	
	telbivudine (Tyzeka)	
	peginterferon alfa-2a (Pegasys) is indicated for both B and C.	

4. Radiating chest burning or pain and an acid taste in the mouth.
5. Diethylpropion and phentermine: adrenergic pathways.

   Dextroamphetamine, methamphetamine: norepinephrine and dopaminergic pathways. Orlistat prevents fat in the diet from being hydrolyzed and absorbed.

Dispensing Medications

1. OTC drugs to treat GERD: Alterna Gel, Gaviscon Extra Strength, Maalox, Mylanta, Phillips Milk of Magnesia, Tagamet HB, Pepcid AC, Axid AR, Zantac 75, Prilosec OTC, Pepcid Complete, Zegerid.
2. Drug companies can change the ingredients in OTC products without having to go through the FDA. This is frequently done to capitalize on a product name and increase sales.
3. Hepatitis A, B, and C; A and B; healthcare workers, HIV+, alcoholics, and children are at risk for, or more likely to contract, hepatitis.
4. Male: $50 + (2.3 \times 15) = 84.5$ kg.
5. Female: $45.5 + (2.3 \times 6) = 59.3$ kg.
6. $\text{BMI} = (200/2.2)/(66 \times 2.5/100)^2 = 33.4$.

Internet Research

1. This exercise reinforces the concept of clinical trials, which was introduced in Chapter 1, and helps to illustrate the different types of methods and conclusions that correspond to each of the three phases. The National Library of Medicine indexes trials that are currently recruiting patients on its clinical trials site (www.clinicaltrials.gov) and lists the location, phase, and drug being tested. In addition, the Crohn's and Colitis Foundation of America (CCFA) (www.ccfa.org) indexes clinical trials related to Crohn's disease and ulcerative colitis.
2. The student's response should include peptic ulcer and may differentiate between stomach and intestinal (duodenal) ulcers. Nonulcerative dyspepsia and "other" stomach concerns may also be included in the student's answer, though not all sites include these disorders. Internet sources include the Helicobacter Foundation (www.helico.com) and the National Institute of Diabetes and Digestive and Kidney Diseases of the National Institutes of Health (www.niddk.nih.gov).

Reflecting on the Profession

1. Students may discuss flash cards and practice quizzes (both of which are available on the Study Guide CD) as well as charting diseases with recommended treatments and small-group review. Encourage them to share ideas.
2. This is an opportunity for students to apply prior work and volunteer experiences and project participation to their thinking about their chosen field.

What Would You Do?

1. Get immune globulin (IG) right away.
2. It's okay, as a pharmacy technician, to read the small print to the patient, but you cannot make a recommendation. Get the pharmacist to help her.

Chapter 11 Renal System Drugs

Pharmaceuticals and Body Functions

Multiple Choice

1. b
2. a

3. b
4. b
5. c
6. b
7. d
8. a
9. b
10. c

True/False

1. false, blue-green
2. false, Hytrin has a longer half-life
3. false, could cause aluminum toxicity
4. false, four
5. false, treats end-stage renal disease
6. false, they do need iron to replenish stores in the bone marrow
7. true
8. true
9. false, Elmiron
10. true

Diseases and Drug Therapies

1. Filtration: substances leave the blood in the glomerulus.

   Secretion: hydrogen ions, potassium ions, weak acids, and weak bases are secreted.

   Excretion: process of eliminating waste material.

   Reabsorption: substances selectively pulled back into the blood.
2. Iron is needed to replenish iron stores in bone marrow. Folic acid is needed for erythropoiesis.
3. Loss of renal reserve, renal insufficiency, chronic renal failure, end-stage renal disease.
4. Urispas exerts a direct spasmolytic effect on smooth muscle, primarily in the urinary tract, acts on the detrusor muscle, increases bladder capacity, and also has local anesthetic and analgesic effects.

   Pro-Banthine competitively blocks the action of acetylcholine at postganglionic parasympathetic receptor sites.

5.

Thiazide Diuretics	Loop Diuretics	Potassium-Sparing Diuretics	Osmotic Diuretics	Carbonic Anhydrase Inhibitors	Miscellaneous Diuretics
Esidrix	Bumex	Midamor	Osmitrol	Diamox	Lozol
Enduron	Edecrin	Aldactone		Neptazane	Zaroxolyn
	Lasix	Dyrenium			
	Demadex	Inspra			

Dispensing Medications

1. John Doe, 4 mL

   Priscilla Perkins, 2 mL

   Peter Pumpkin, 3 mL

   No, there is 11 mL total.
2. Belinda Bold (date)

   Macrodantin 50 mg #80

   Take two capsules four times daily until all are taken.

   Refills #4 Dr. J. Bland

   Attach a "Take with FOOD" sticker.
3. 168 folic acid (3 tablets/day × 7 days/week × 8 weeks)

   60 B_6

Internet Research

1. The prostate screening test is performed through a PSA (prostate specific antigen) test. An elevated level of PSA alerts the physician to the potential for cancer. However, the presence of BHP will also raise the level of PSA. Moreover, BHP symptoms are similar to those of prostate cancer. Consequently, a biopsy is needed to verify the screening test results. This test can find cancer before it spreads, offering a better chance for cure. The American Cancer Society (www.cancer.org) is the definitive source of information on cancer screening and provides an excellent overview of the PSA test.

2. By flushing excess water and sodium from the body, diuretics reduce the amount of fluid in the blood. In turn, the pressure in the vessel is reduced. The National Heart, Lung, and Blood Institute of the National Institutes of Health (www.nhlbi.nih.gov) is a good source of information on blood pressure control.

Reflecting on the Profession

1. Students may discuss flash cards and practice quizzes (both of which are available on the Study Guide CD) as well as sketching the renal system and small-group review. Encourage them to share ideas.
2. This is another opportunity for students to reflect on the balance between empathy and professional detachment. Encourage them to discuss any experiences they have had with pain management.

What Would You Do?

1. Make sure the pharmacist is aware of this interaction. Also note whether it is the same prescriber who is prescribing both drugs. If it is the same prescriber, then it is the prescriber's responsibility to do the appropriate tests. Even though, theoretically, patients should not need potassium, in real life they often do.
2. This is debatable. It is a fact, and does not involve the pharmacist's judgment. This color change is going to happen no matter what, but because it involves ingestion of the medication, it probably would be best to refrain from discussing it with the patient. However, the technician could emphasize the importance of the patient reading the literature that accompanies the medication.

Chapter 12 Drugs for Cardiovascular Diseases

Pharmaceuticals and Body Functions

Multiple Choice

1. c
2. a
3. b
4. c
5. a
6. b
7. d
8. b
9. c
10. b

True/False

1. false, nitroglycerin
2. false, take patch off while sleeping
3. false, reduce side effects
4. false, will not dissolve a clot
5. false, 30%
6. true
7. false, it is used as an antiarrhythmic
8. true
9. true
10. false, angiotensin I–converting enzyme

Matching

1. b
2. c
3. c
4. c
5. b
6. a
7. a
8. b
9. a
10. a
11. b
12. b
13. a
14. b
15. b
16. c
17. a
18. a
19. c
20. b

Diseases and Drug Therapies

1. Two of each of the following groups:

   membrane-stabilizing agents: quinidine, procainamide, disopyramide, moricizine, lidocaine, mexiletine, phenytoin, tocainide, flecainide.

Beta blockers: acebutolol, esmolol, propranolol, sotalol.

Potassium channel blockers: amiodarone, dofetilide.

Calcium channel blockers: verapamil, diltiazem.

2. Step 1. change lifestyle

   Step 2. monotherapy

   Step 3. add diuretic if not already taking

   Step 4. add third drug

3. Anticoagulants prevent clots from forming: Angiomax, argatroban, Arixtra, Coumadin, Fragmin, heparin, Innohep, Lovenox, Refludan.

   Fibrinolytics dissolve clots already formed: Abbokinase, Activase, Retavase, Streptase, TNKase.

4.

HMG-CoA Reductase Inhibitors	Fibric Acid Derivatives	Bile Acid Sequestrants	Misc.	Combination
Zocor	clofibrate (no brand name) TriLipex, Fibricor	Questran	Zetia Lovaza	Caduet
Crestor				Advicor
Pravachol	Lopid	Colestid	Niacor	Simcor
Altocor, Mevacor	TriCor	WelChol		Provigard PAC Vytorin
Lescol			Fiberall, Metamucil	
Lipitor, Livalo				

Dispensing Medications

1. 90 doses
2. 30 mg would be a better dosage.

   1 mg protamine sulfate to 90–120 units heparin, so 3,000 divided by 100 equals 30
3. Yes, these drugs are synergistic.

Internet Research

1. This exercise requires that the student understand the different manifestations of heart disease. You might want to point out that these three populations will generally overlap significantly. Because myocardial infarction is an event as opposed to a condition, prevalence data cannot be assigned to it. This distinction may help to reinforce the concepts of prevalence and incidence. The American Heart Association (http://www.americanheart.org) is a good source of heart disease statistics.

2. Comparison of Low-Molecular-Weight Heparins

Drug	Indications
dalteparin (Fragmin)	Prophylaxis of DVT in orthopedic and abdominal surgery
	Prophylaxis of thromboembolism in general surgery
	Treatment of DVT
	Treatment of unstable angina and non-Q-wave myocardial infarction (given with aspirin)
	Anticoagulation in hemodialysis (HD) and hemofiltration
enoxaparin (Lovenox)	Prophylaxis of DVT in orthopedic and abdominal surgery
	Treatment of DVT with or without pulmonary embolism, when given with warfarin
	Prevention of ischemic complications of unstable angina and non-Q-wave MI when given with aspirin

Drug	Indications
	Prophylaxis of thromboembolism in high risk abdominal, gynecological, or urological surgeries or colorectal surgery
tinzaparin (Innohep)	Prophylaxis of thromboembolism in orthopedic surgery
	Prophylaxis of thromboembolism in general surgery
	Treatment of DVT and pulmonary embolism

Reflecting on the Profession

1. This is another opportunity to explore empathy and professionalism.
2. Point students toward the online materials on professionalism, and recommend that they spend some time with one or more books on the subject. Encourage students to discuss the kinds of skills they possess and creative ideas for presenting them.

What Would You Do?

1. Encourage the patient to discuss this with the pharmacist or prescriber, but above all not to quit taking the medication until he has done so. This would not be counseling. Telling patients to take their medication as prescribed is not counseling—it is simply following the prescriber's directions. If you thought you could tell a patient to "take it every other day" or something like that, that would be counseling. It could be very dangerous to deviate from a prescriber's directions or for the patient to stop taking the blood pressure medication. It would not be wise for the technician to go into the reasons (saying "you might have a stroke," or something similar), but to tell patients, whatever they do, not to stop taking their medications would not be counseling and could save someone's life.
2. It is okay to make the patient aware of the fact that he can get bottles of #25 and that, once the bottle is opened, the beyond use date becomes effective and he will have to reorder at that time whether he has 100 or 25. Cutting drug costs is an area in which technicians can play a critical role, and patients will be most appreciative. This has nothing to do with taking the drug.

Chapter 13 Drugs for Muscle and Joint Disease and Pain

Pharmaceuticals and Body Functions

Multiple Choice

1. b
2. d
3. b
4. c
5. a
6. a
7. d
8. b
9. a
10. a

True/False

1. false, have not
2. true
3. false, short-term
4. false, indomethacin and ketorolac
5. false, colchicine
6. false, acts peripherally
7. true
8. true
9. false, 1,200 is maximum dose/day
10. false, diclofenac, flurbiprofen, ketorolac

Diseases and Drug Therapies

1. Block release of ACh, prevent destruction of ACh, prevent ACh from reaching receptors, agents that bind to ACh receptors
2. The major metabolite of Soma is meprobamate, which is addictive.
3. Ophthalmics: diclofenac, flurbiprofen, ketorolac
   OTCs: ibuprofen, ketoprofen, naproxen
   IV: indomethacin, ketorolac.

4. Suppository: indomethacin
   Patch: diclofenac
   IM: ketorolac
   Topical: diclofenac.
5. Ultram binds to opiate receptors and inhibits reuptake of norepinephrine and serotonin. It acts centrally.
6. Morning stiffness; joint tenderness; sterile turbid synovial fluid; X-ray changes; presence of rheumatoid factor; soft tissue swelling of the first joint, second within three months.

Dispensing Medications

1. Peptic ulcer patients, gout patients, patients on oral anticoagulants, patients with clotting disorders, patients at risk of Reye's syndrome, patients intolerant to aspirin.
2. a. Cataflam: eyedrop
   b. Ansaid: po
   c. Indocin: IV
   d. Indocin: suppository
   e. Toradol: IM
3. 0.5 to 1 mg/mL in preservative-free sterile water.

Internet Research

1. This exercise will help to reinforce the differences among these common OTC analgesics. The student should list two or three contraindications for each drug and three to five side effects. Indications should include:

   Aspirin: pain or fever, arthritis, preventing heart attack or stroke.

   Acetaminophen: pain and fever.

   Ibuprofen: arthritis; tendinitis; menstrual cramps; sprains, strains or other injuries

   The National Library of Medicine lists drugs alphabetically on its MedlinePlus site (http://medlineplus.gov). YourHealth.com (www.yourhealth.com) also covers this topic.
2. This exercise reinforces the concept of clinical trials, which was introduced in Chapter 1, and helps to illustrate the different types of methods and conclusions that correspond to each of the three phases. The National Library of Medicine indexes trials that are currently recruiting patients on its clinical trials site (www.clinicaltrials.gov) and lists the location, phase, and drug being tested. The National Institute of Arthritis and Musculoskeletal and Skin Diseases (NIAMS) (www.niams.nih.gov) also indexes information on clinical trials related to arthritis.

Reflecting on the Profession

1. This is another opportunity to share personal experiences, explore empathy, and discuss professionalism.
2. Any student who has interviewed should reflect on what went well and what didn't, then apply those experiences to thinking about interviewing for a pharm tech position. Online research as well as the electronic resources included with this course can help students explore the topic more fully.

What Would You Do?

1. Nothing says the medication guide has to be attached by the pharmacist. It might even be a good idea to assign this task to the technician. It would just be important that the right guide goes with the right drug class, or drug. You might want to check with the pharmacist and see how he or she wants to handle this.
2. Call the prescriber; you cannot fill the prescription because the strength is not indicated.

Chapter 14 Hormonal Disorders and Their Treatment

Pharmaceuticals and Body Functions

Multiple Choice

1. b
2. a
3. a
4. c
5. d
6. c
7. a
8. c
9. a
10. d

True/False

1. true
2. true
3. true
4. true
5. false, hCG
6. false, a.m.
7. true
8. false, hyperglycemia, long-term; hypoglycemia, short-term
9. false, they do
10. false, should not

Diseases and Drug Therapies

1. Positive effects: eases transition into menopause, prevents bone loss.

   Side effects: hypercoagulability, glucose intolerance, fluid retention, weight gain, bloating, breast tenderness, mild nausea and vomiting, some cancers, increased risk of MI.
2. Increased urination, thirst, hunger, weight loss, easily fatigued, irritability, nausea and vomiting, ketoacidosis, visual changes, glycosuria, numbness and tingling, slow wound healing, frequent infections, nocturia.
3. Patients with migraines, mild hypertension, thrombosis history, endometriosis, chronic cystic mastitis, breast cancer, stroke, MI, and smoking.
4. Levothyroxine: Synthroid, Levoxyl (T_4), thyroid hormone replacement.

   PTU: blocks synthesis of thyroid

   methimazole: Tapazole, returns the hyperthyroid patient to a normal state prior to thyroidectomy.
5. Deficiency of endogenous hormone, malnutrition, systemic illness, endocrine deficiency, psychosocial stress.
6. d
7. c
8. b
9. a
10. a
11. a
12. b
13. b
14. a

Dispensing Medications

1. The patient must be counseled to take the drug 30 minutes before the first meal of the day, with a full glass of water, and to not lie down for 30 minutes after taking it to avoid esophageal burning.
2. Patient is gestational diabetic; birth control pills are contraindicated.
3. The patient can be informed that the insulin is safe outside the refrigerator for 28 days.
4. Patient 1: 35 units x 90 = 3,150

   1,000 units per box

   4 boxes

   Patient 2: 55 units x 30 = 1,600

   1,000 units per box

   2 boxes

   Patient 3: Humalog 35 x 90 = 3,150

   Lantus 25 x 90 = 2,250

   1,000 units per box

   4 Humalog

   3 Lantus

Internet Research

1. Who is at risk: women over age 65; women with low calcium intake, low body weight, or family history.

   How diagnosed: through computed tomography (CT) and ultrasound.

   Those listed in the risk population should be screened.

   Internet source: The National Osteoporosis Foundation (http://www.nof.org).
2. This exercise asks the student to evaluate the quality and utility of information provided by various websites for a particular audience, the patient. The student may observe that some sites are more oriented toward the medical professional and do not provide enough background or practical information for the patient. The student may also observe that certain sites are easier to navigate than others and that certain sites have more comprehensive coverage, catering to patients who know very little about their disease and only want practical tips as well as those who seek a greater depth of understanding. Internet sources include the American Diabetes Association (http://www.

diabetes.org) and the Joslin Diabetes Center (http://www.joslin.harvard.edu).

Reflecting on the Profession

1. Students may discuss flash cards and practice quizzes (both of which are available on the Study Guide CD) as well as charting the hormone system, its diseases and medications, and other uses. Encourage them to share ideas in class and in small-group review sessions.
2. Students should discuss issues like ethics, nonjudgmentalism, maintaining professional behavior, privacy, and public safety. If a student expresses reservations, encourage discussion, but don't let debate slide into arguments over religion or morality.

What Would You Do?

1. Obviously something is going on here; make the pharmacist aware. That is about all you can really do. If you take it up with his parents, would that be a HIPAA violation? (He is under age.) Basically, it is going to depend on the philosophy of the pharmacist who is in charge that night as to how it will be handled. Once you have made the proper person aware, you have fulfilled your obligation and done your job.
2. The morning after pill is simply a very large dose of oral contraceptive. Explain this to the technician, and perhaps ask the pharmacist to step in to discuss the issue with the technician.

Chapter 15 Topical, Ophthalmic, and Otic Medications

Pharmaceuticals and Body Functions

Multiple Choice

1. a
2. c
3. b
4. c
5. c
6. d
7. a
8. d
9. d
10. a

True/False

1. false, the statement describes impetigo
2. false, the statement describes erysipelas
3. false, the statement describes folliculitis
4. false, boils are furuncles
5. false, the exception is Psorcon
6. true
7. false, eyedrops for the ear, never eardrops in the eye
8. false, it is a steroid
9. false, it is an eardrop
10. false, only suspensions should be used

Diseases and Drug Therapies

1. Fungicide: anything that destroys fungi.

   Disinfectant: chemicals applied to nonliving material.

   Germicide: anything that destroys bacteria but not necessarily spores.

   Antiseptic: chemicals applied to living tissue for the purpose of killing bacteria or inhibiting their growth.
2. Odor, taste, and staining quality.
3. Acne is caused by increased gland activity at puberty. A lesion begins with a plugged terminal sebaceous duct. A layer of dirt may then be picked up. The gland and hair follicle become engorged with sebum to form a papule. If the contents become infected, it turns into a pustule surrounded by an inflamed area. Treatment options include UV light, Retin-A, Differin, erythromycin, tetracycline, and Azelex.
4. Periactin, Benadryl, Seldane
5. They have the ability to penetrate through the skin; thus, they can suppress the hypothalamus-pituitary axis. They can also cause skin eruptions, burning sensation, atropic striae, and petechiae.
6. bimatoprost (Latisse)
7. 0.015%

Dispensing Medications

1. Lindane; Nix, Elimite, Rid Mousse (see Table 15.7)

2. Lotrimin or Monistat
3. Wash hands.
   Shake container.
   Remove cap.
   Tilt head.
   Pull lower eyelid down.
   Hold tip directly over eye.
   Look up, place a drop in pocket formed by lower lid.
   Release eyelid.
   Wait 5 or 10 minutes before applying any other medication to eye.
   Replace cap.
   Wash hands.

Internet Research

1. Preschool and elementary school children and their families constitute the primary risk population for head lice. Girls and women are at greater risk. Head lice are rare in African Americans. Common signs and symptoms include a feeling of something moving in the hair, itching caused by a reaction to the bites, irritability, and sores on the head. The National Pediculosis Association sponsors a site called HeadLice.org (http://www.headlice.org) that covers this topic in depth. The Centers for Disease Control (http://www.cdc.gov) also covers this topic.
2. This exercise will help the student develop a more thorough understanding of the different components of the research and development process. The Glaucoma Research Foundation (http://www.glaucoma.org) has a comprehensive site with an emphasis on patient education and research. The American Academy of Ophthalmology (AAO) (http://www.aao.org) also indexes glaucoma-related research programs.

Reflecting on the Profession

1. Students should note that it is okay to direct a customer to the correct shelf, identify active ingredients, read instructions, or identify different flavor options, but that advising the customer on which medication might be best for him or her is the pharmacist's responsibility.
2. Students should be encouraged to consider their doubts and misgivings, if any. Students can also support one another.

What Would You Do?

1. You must bring this to the attention of the director. Order as much as possible in unit dose; more and more manufacturers are putting eyedrops into unit dose packing so that it cannot be used on multiple patients. But this is a very real problem that occurs every day where there is an ophthalmic clinic.
2. Make the pharmacist aware of the situation. The patient is underage, so it is okay to let the parent know. This really would be a judgment call though; it would be best to let the pharmacist make the decision.

Unit 4 Chemotherapy and Miscellaneous Pharmaceutical Products

Chapter 16 Recombinant Drugs and Chemotherapy

Pharmaceuticals and Body Functions

Multiple Choice

1. a
2. b
3. a
4. d
5. d
6. a
7. d
8. d
9. d
10. a

True/False

1. true
2. true

3. false, do not shake
4. true
5. true
6. false, inhibits viral replication
7. false, t-cells
8. false, interferon
9. false, antibiotics
10. true

Diseases and Drug Therapies

1. Limited sources, small quantities, unsure purity.
2. Skin and mucous membranes; nonspecific defense; immune response.
3. In remission the tumor is in an inactive period during which there is no cell division and growth. The disease is not cured, but the patient has more time.
4. Resistance is lack of responsiveness of the cancer cells to chemotherapy.
5.

MAb	Target	Source
abciximab	cardiovascular	combination
alemtuzumab	miscellaneous	human
daclizumab	immune	human
gemtuzumab	miscellaneous	human
ibritumomab	miscellaneous	mouse

Dispensing Medications

1. Have pharmacist notify the doctor regarding limiting use to five years.
2. The prescriber needs to be contacted to clarify the prescription, because several different ingredients can be used. The prescriber should also confirm that the ingredients should be mixed in equal parts.

Internet Research

1. The heart, kidney, and liver are the three most commonly transplanted organs. Other organs commonly transplanted include the lung, bone marrow, and pancreas. The American Heart Association (http://www.americanheart.org) has good information on heart transplants. The National Kidney Foundation (NKF) (http://www.kidney.org) covers kidney transplants, and the American Liver Foundation (ALF) (http://www.liverfoundation.org) covers liver transplants.
2. This exercise will introduce the student to new chemotherapeutics and reinforce the importance of drug research and testing. It requires the student to distinguish between chemotherapy research and other types of cancer treatment research (e.g., radiotherapies, brachytherapies, photodynamic therapies). Internet sources include the American Institute for Cancer Research (http://www.aicr.org) and the Alpha Cancer Information Resource, the Educational Resource of the Coalition of National Cancer Cooperative Groups (http://www.alphacancer.com).

Reflecting on the Profession

1. Students should discuss attention to detail, thorough knowledge of steps and processes, not rushing, and the value of practice and training.
2. Role playing is one great way to practice professionalism. Consider pairing students up for a role playing exercise, then assign roles for each. Remember to give students an opportunity to be on both sides of the pharmacy counter. Also, encourage students to draw on previous experiences.

What Would You Do?

1. Someone must be notified to correct this situation for this patient. It could be very dangerous not to mention the discomfort for the patient to undergo this treatment without the pre-meds (acetaminophen and diphenhydramine) and hydration.
2. Throw it away and start over; you can't take the chance.

Chapter 17 Vitamins, OTC Supplements, Antidotes, and Miscellaneous Topics

Pharmaceuticals and Body Functions

Multiple Choice

1. c
2. a
3. a
4. d

5. d
6. d
7. c
8. c
9. d
10. b

True/False

1. true
2. true
3. true
4. false, same
5. false, recommended for memory loss, cerebral insufficiency, peripheral vascular insufficiency
6. true
7. false, chamomile
8. false, ginkgo
9. false, there are
10. true

Diseases and Drug Therapies

1. Three of the following: poor wound healing, infections, anemia, specific GI disease and/or hypermetabolic states, failure to tolerate enteral nutrition.
2. Hyperglycemia or hypoglycemia, dehydration, liver toxicity, elevated serum triglycerides, high serum lipid concentrations, hypoalbuminemia, hyperammonemia, acid-base imbalance, failure to induce anabolism, imbalance of electrolytes.
3. Hotline: 1-800-222-1222.
4. The authors realize that the section on alternative medicine may be controversial. The primary source used was "Natural Medicines Comprehensive Data Base." We believe it is as good as anything out there on this subject. Because there are very few good evidence-based studies on these drugs, there will be many differing opinions. The official alternative medicine site of the U.S. government is the National Center for Complementary and Alternative Medicine at http://nccam.nih.gov.
   1) yohimbe
   2) echinacea
   3) ginger
   4) melatonin
   5) saw palmetto
5. 1-c
   2-b
   3-d
   4-e
   5-a

Dispensing Medications

1. flumazenil (Romazicon) and naloxone (Narcan)
2. epinephrine, antihistamine, and IV hydrocortisone

Internet Research

1. The students' answers will vary depending on their source. They should include at least five tips for prevention. Instructions for dealing with a case of suspected poisoning should include the following points: (1) call a poison control center or 911, and (2) seek medical advice about whether or not to induce vomiting. A plethora of sites cover this topic; the American Association of Poison Control Centers (http://www.aapcc.org) is a good one.
2. The challenge of this exercise is for the student to ferret out clinically appropriate information from among all the "hype" that has proliferated on the Web. There are good sites out there, including the Herbage Guide to Herbs (http://www.herbweb.com), Medherb.com (http://www.medherb.com), and Botanical.com's Modern Herbal site (http://www.botanical.com). You may want to lead a class discussion centered on the regulatory issues surrounding herbal medicines, e.g., "Is it a good or bad idea to regulate these products?"

Reflecting on the Profession

1. This is an opportunity for students to think critically about the spacing and management of a pharmacy and how they would work in that environment. There are no right or wrong answers.
2. Handling oneself in a crisis could be key to a pharm tech's work; encourage students to explore their feelings and concerns on this issue.

What Would You Do?

1. Students' answers will vary.

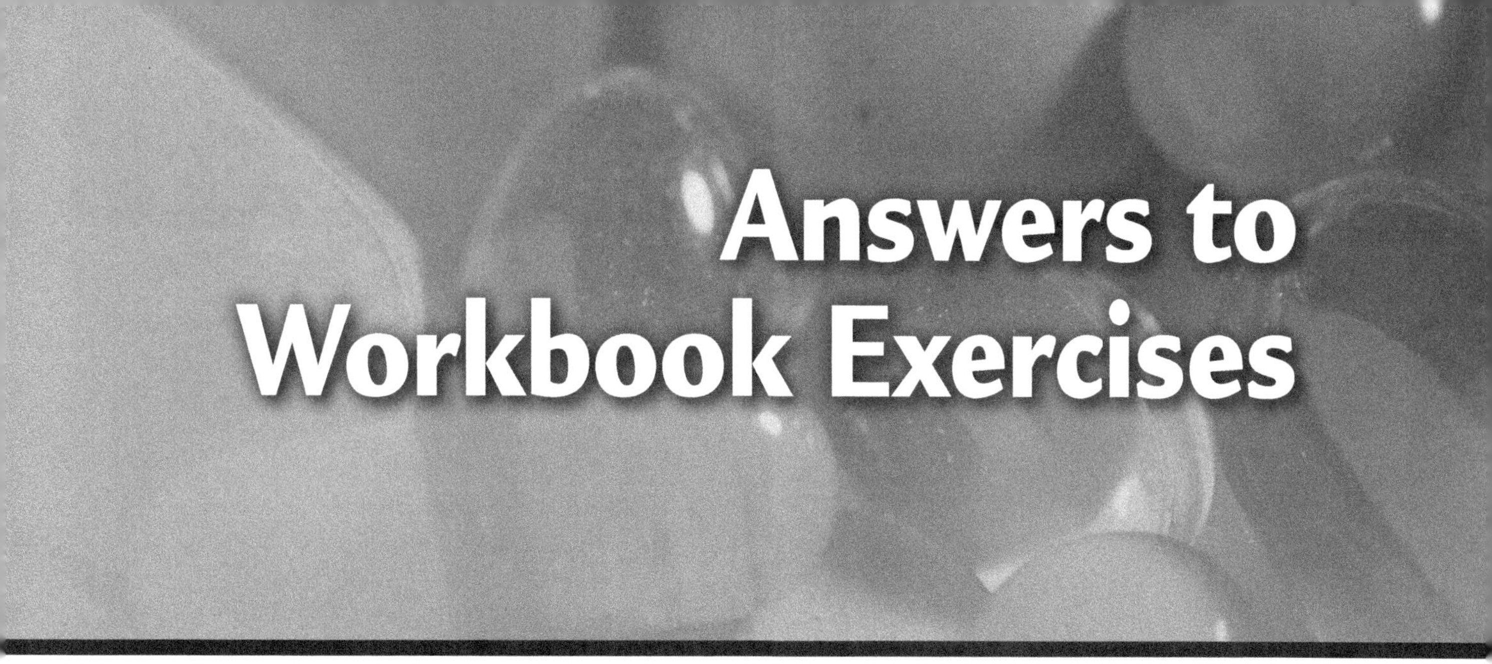

Answers to Workbook Exercises

Unit 1 Introduction to Pharmacology

Chapter 1 Evolution of Medicinal Drugs

Understanding Pharmacology and Pharmacokinetics

1. Two pioneers of chemical sterilization in the healthcare setting are Ignaz Philip Semmelweis who discovered that the use of chlorinated lime water in maternity wards decreased the spread of puerperal fever, and Joseph Lister who introduced the use of carbolic acid in sterilization of surgical equipment.
2. Pharmacists should perform tasks b and e. Technicians should be responsible for tasks a, c, and d.
3. The American Association of Pharmacy Technicians
4. Don Ballington; PTEC was organized for pharmacy technician educators to focus on sharing ideas. Paradigm published the first Pharmacology text for technicians.
5. USP (1820), APhA (1852), FDA (1927), DEA (1973)
6. This clinical trial is in phase I, because researchers are recruiting a small number of healthy people to study what happens to the drug in the human body.
7. The Journal of Pharmacy Technology
8. the body's humors: blood, yellow bile, black bile, and phlegm
9. NSAIDS and antidepressants
10. A vaccine is a prophylactic drug, because it prevents disease. A vaccine does not treat disease.
11. placebo
12. X
13. *Orange Book*
14. OTC
15. two
16. generic
17. MedWatch
18. *Dispensatorium*
19. Massachusetts Medical Society
20. salts
21. minute
22. New Drug Application (NDA)
23. controlled substances
24. Sir Frederick Banting and Charles Best
25. double blind

Matching–Terms and Definitions

26. n
27. s
28. m
29. l
30. k

31. j
32. h
33. g
34. c
35. d
36. e
37. f
38. p
39. q
40. r
41. t
42. y
43. x
44. z
45. w
46. u
47. v
48. a
49. b
50. o

Puzzling the Technician–Terms and Definitions

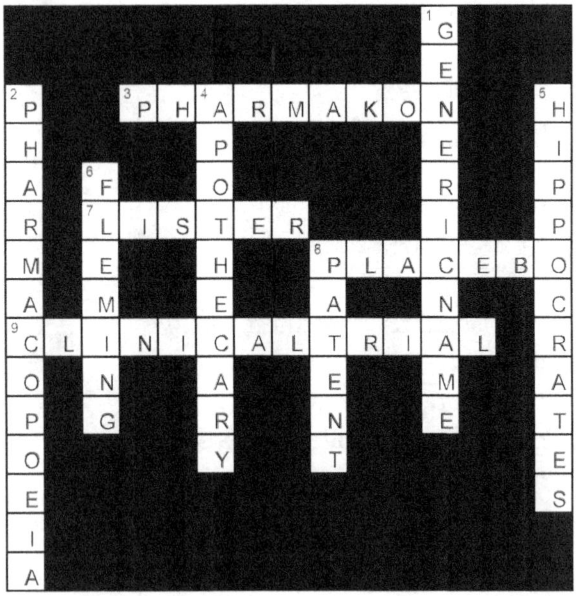

Chapter 2 Basic Concepts of Pharmacology

Understanding Pharmacology and Pharmacokinetics

1. The drug is an agonist because it triggered a response similar to the action of the body's own chemical messengers.
2. The goal is to produce in the body a response that cures or controls a specific disease or medical condition.
3. The body acts to maintain homeostasis to keep the body's living processes in balance.
4. The drug has a local effect because it must be applied to each affected nail.
5. Using lower doses and having increased efficacy is categorized as synergy.
6. The two types of drug inhibition are: a) competitive - two drugs may inhibit or enhance metabolism of each other when given together; b) noncompetitive inhibition - one drug totally blocks enzyme activity and impairs metabolism.
7. Because Mrs. Holly is not seeking the use of Oxycontin for euphoria, she is dependent on the drug for prevention of cancer-related pain.
8. The loading dose will rapidly bring the blood concentration to a therapeutic level. The first two tablets are the loading dose.
9. Idiosyncratic
10. Because drug B is dosed less often, it has the longer duration of action. The free level will be 1.5 mcg/mL × 15 mcg/mL × 0.9 = 13.5 mcg; 15 mcg − 13.5 mcg = 1.5 mcg/mL.
11. A half-life is the amount of time it takes for the body to eliminate half of the original concentration of a drug from the body. Five to seven half-lives are necessary to eliminate nearly all of a drug from the body.
12. blood-brain barrier
13. trough
14. clearance
15. absorption
16. longer
17. bioavailability
18. therapeutic range
19. 5

Matching–Terms and Definitions

20. b
21. d
22. e
23. f
24. o
25. p
26. q
27. ee
28. g
29. n
30. y
31. h
32. m
33. r
34. t
35. s
36. u
37. i
38. v
39. w
40. z
41. aa
42. j
43. a
44. l
45. cc
46. bb
47. c
48. dd
49. x
50. z

Puzzling the Technician–Terms and Definitions

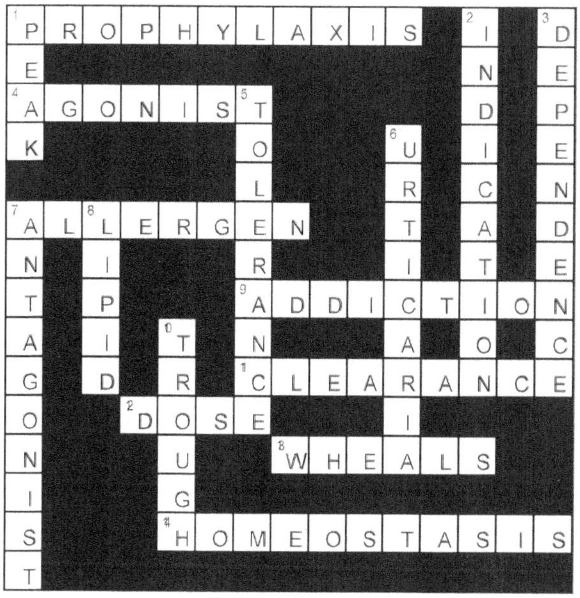

Chapter 3 Dispensing Medications

Understanding Pharmacology and Pharmacokinetics

1. Sublingual nitroglycerin enters the bloodstream directly from the membrane of the mouth and produces its effects more quickly than nitroglycerin that is swallowed.
2. Children and the elderly; Aging among the elderly affects how medications work in their bodies and they more commonly face chronic diseases. Children undergo such rapid growth that dosage and treatment decisions can be quite tricky.
3. rectal route
4. Prescriptions are generally good for only one year; those for C-IIIs and C-IVs are for only six months.
5. No, it is too old.
6. A protocol must be in place; flu shots do not require a prescription, but there must be a protocol in place authorized by an MD.
7. The patient can't throw it up, and the body absorbs the medication faster.

8. Some drugs on both lists include: amitriptyline (Elavil), reserine, dipyridamole (Persantine), thioridazine (Mellaril), chlorpromazine (Thorazine), clorazepate (Tranxene), diazepam (Valium), chlordiazepoxide (Librium), and indomethacin (Indocin).
9. Sig or signa
10. Medication Guide
11. Parenteral
12. Topical
13. It reduces errors and improves patient safety by a. eliminating illegible handwriting, b. checking for allergies, c. checking for interactions, d. checking dosing levels, and e. preventing therapeutic duplications.
14. Often, prescriptions do not scan clearly into the computer system and they are hard to read. The original is always clearer.
15. Compliance
16. Antigens
17. Mast cells
18. H_2
19. Dilation
20. Medication

Matching–Terms and Definitions

21. p
22. a
23. o
24. w
25. r
26. c
27. d
28. e
29. f
30. g
31. n
32. m
33. l
34. k
35. i
36. h
37. bb
38. ee
39. y
40. z
41. s
42. t
43. v
44. u
45. dd
46. q
47. cc
48. b
49. x
50. j
51. aa

Puzzling the Technician–Terms and Definitions

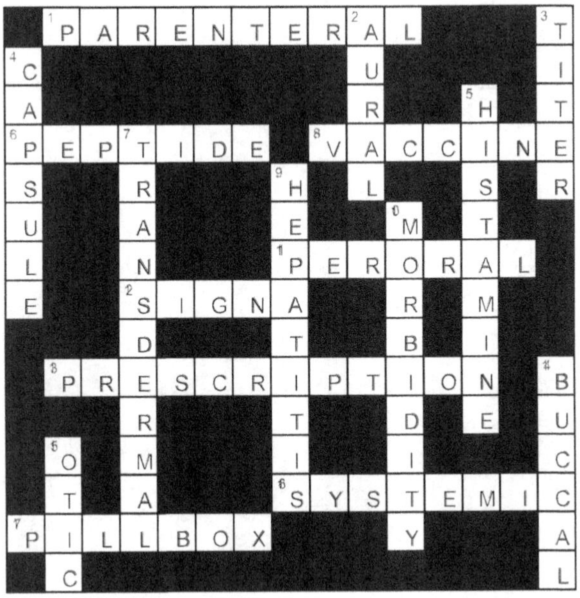

Unit 2 Major Classes of Pharmaceutical Products I

Chapter 4 Antibiotics

Reading Drug Labels and Medication Orders

1. a. Because 250 mg/5 mL is prescribed and 125 mg/5 mL is available, it would take 2 tsp (or 10 mL) of 125 mg/5 mL to equal 1 tsp (or 5 mL) of 250 mg/5 mL. The instructions will read, "Take 2 teaspoonsful (10 mL) 3 times a day for 7 days."
   b. 10 mL/dose × 3 doses/day × 7 days/treatment = 210 mL/treatment
   c. 250 mg/5 mL × 5 mL/1 tsp × 3 tsp/day = 750 mg/day
2. penicillin
3. a. Take one tablet twice a day for three days.
   b. 2 tablets/day × 3 days/treatment = 6 tablets/treatment
4. 400 mg × 1 mL/40mg = 10 mL
5. amoxicillin
6. Unless otherwise noted, a concentration of 13.6% means 13.6 g/100 mL. Therefore, to determine the amount of milligrams in 10 mL, x mg/10 mL = 13,600 mg/100 mL, x mg = 1360 mg.
7. 100 mg × 0.1 mL/2.25 mg = 4.44 mL; 4.44 mL − 1 mL (drug solution) = 3.4 mL NS. (*Note:* The calculation takes into account that the100 mg solution already had a volume of 1 mL.)
8. a. 285 mg/dose × 5 mL/75 mg = 19 mL/dose. The label should read, "Take 19 mL by mouth every 8 hours for a total of 3 doses per day."
   b. 100 mL/bottle × 1 dose/19 mL = 5.26 doses
9. 2,000,000 units/50 mL = 40,000 units/mL; 1,200,000 units × 1 mL/40,000 units = 30 mL
10. a. Take 1 capsule by mouth 2 times a day for 14 days.
    b. 2 capsules/day × 14 days = 28 capsules

Understanding the Larger Medical Context

11. The patient receives a large first dose and subsequent doses are usually one half of the first dose.
12. a. Minocycline can cause photosensitivity in patients. Timmy could use a sunscreen to manage this side effect.
    b. Timmy should not take minocycline with antacids or laxatives.
13. Take two tablets now, then one tablet daily for a total of five days. This medication should be taken with food.
14. amoxicillin
    amoxicillin-clavulanate (Augmentin)
    ampicillin
    cefadroxil (Duricef)
    cefaclor (Ceclor)
    cefpodoxim (Vantin)
    cefprozil (Cefzil)
    ceftibutin (Cedax)
    cephalexin (Keflex)
    loracarbef (Lorabid)
    penicillin
15. vancomycin
16. metronidazole (Flagyl)
17. Cefepime is the only fourth-generation cephalosporin.
18. Because they cover a wide range of organisms.

Dispensing and Storing Drugs

19. at room temperature
20. in the refrigerator
21 at room temperature
22. at room temperature
23. in the refrigerator
24. in the refrigerator
25. in the refrigerator
26. at room temperature
27. in the refrigerator
28. at room temperature

Putting Safety First

29. Not mg, the dose would be 2 grams (g)
30. Zithromax 500 mg dose is recommended for dental procedures.
31. Amoxicillin tid is the appropriate dose.
32. Fortaz can be mixed in either NS or D_5W and placed in either a 50 mL or 100 mL bag and administered over 30 minutes.
33. The dose is appropriate.

Understanding Concepts

34. metronidazole (Flagyl)
35. The signa should read "Take 10 milliliters three times a day for 10 days." Filling the prescription will take three bottles, and the medicine will be fruit flavored.
36. Call the dentist and suggest changing the drug.
37. Penicillin or amoxacillin (2 grams), clindamyacin (600 mg), or azithromycin (500 mg).
38. Medication Guides
    ciprofloxacin (Cipro)
    gemifloxacin (Factive)
    levofloxacin (Levaquin)
    moxifloxacin (Avelox)
    norfloxacin (Noroxin)
    ofloxacin (Floxin)
    telithromycin (Ketek)
    Note: Most are the quinolones.
39. Black Box Warnings are required for the following drugs in this chapter:
    clindamycin (Cleocin)
    metronidazole (Flagyl)
    neomycin (Neo-Fradin)
    penicillin G
    streptomycin
    tindazole (Tindamax)
40. linezolid (Zyvox)
41. You would choose the otic (ear) medication. The sig would read "Instill 4 drops in both ears twice daily."
42. For this prescription, you would choose the ophthalmic (eye) medication. The sig would read, "Instill 1 drop in each eye every morning and every evening."
43. The generic for Bactrim DS is sulfamethoxazole-trimethoprim 800/160. The sig would read, "Take one tablet by mouth twice daily for 10 days for UTI." You would dispense 20 tablets. A UTI is a urinary tract infection. After dispensing the medication, you would clean the tray with alcohol.
44. Suggest flavoring the drug with another additive.

Matching–Brand and Generic Drug Names

45. f
46. a
47. b
48. j
49. g
50. h
51. i
52. e
53. d
54. c

Matching–Terms and Definitions

55. b
56. g
57. e
58. i
59. d
60. f
61. j
62. h
63. c
64. a

Chapter 5 Therapy for Fungal and Viral Infections

Reading Drug Labels and Medication Orders

1. a. Amphotericin B cannot be mixed in normal saline because a precipitate may occur. D_5W is the preferred diluent.

b. 60 mg dosed over seven days will be administered, for a total of 420 mg. 420 mg × 1 g/1000 mg = 0.42 g.

c. 420 mg/treatment × 1 vial/50 mg = 8.4 vials for a total dose of 9 vials. However, 14 vials must be used, because amphotericin B is only good for 24 hours per vial after reconstitution.

2. a. The dose is 1 g two times a day times 10 days. 20 doses are in 10 days, or 2 doses/day × 10 days = 20 doses. To determine the number of tablets/dose, 1 g/dose × 1000 mg/1 g = 1000 mg/dose; 1000 mg/dose × 1 caplet/500 mg = 2 caplets/dose. Therefore, there will be 20 doses × 2 caplets/dose = 40 caplets.

   b. Take two caplets by mouth for 10 days.

3. a. 100 mg/dose × 5 mL/50 mg = 10 mL/dose

   b. Since 1 tsp = 5 mL, 10 mL/dose × 1 tsp/5 mL = 2 tsp/dose

   c. Take 2 teaspoonsful (10 mL) by mouth twice daily for 3 days.

   d. 10 mL/dose × 2 doses/day × 3 days/treatment = 60 mL/treatment

4. a. 84 lb × 1 kg/2.2 lb = 38.18 kg; 38.18 kg × 10 mg/kg/dose = 382 mg/dose

   b. 382 mg/dose × 3 doses/day × 1 mL/50 mg = 22.9 mL/day

   c. 100 mL bag

5. Ataripla (efevirenz, emtricitabine, tenofovir), Intelence (etravirine), Norvir (retonavir), Truvada (emtricitabine, tenofovir), Viread (tenofovir)

6. a. Reconstitute with sterile water until the concentration is 20 mg/mL, and then suspend with antacid until the concentration is 10 mg/mL.

   b. 100 mg/dose × 1 mL/10 mg × 2 doses/day = 5 mL/day

   c. 200 mL × day/5 mL = 40 days

7. decreased cost and fewer side effects

8. a. 500 mg/dose × 1 capsule/250 mg × 2 doses/1 day × 30 days/1 month = 120 capsules/month

   b. Ganciclovir is available orally and intravenously, and by intravitreal implant.

9. a. The most likely intended drug is Invirase.

   b. Avoid sunlight. Take with food.

10. a. 1 tsp/dose × 5 mL/tsp × 4 doses/day = 20 mL/day; 60 mL/bottle × 20 mL/day = 3 days/bottle

    b. 1 week × 7 days/week × 1 bottle/3 days = 2.33 bottles. The patient will need 3 bottles.

Understanding the Larger Medical Context

11. Throw it away.
12. Flumadine (rimantadine), Relenza (zanamivir), Symmetrel (Amantadine), Tamiflu (oseltamivir)
13. Sustiva (efavirenz)
14. Rekyataz (atazanavir)
15. tenofovir, efavirenz, emtricitabine

Dispensing and Storing Drugs

16. Epzicom (abacavir/lamivudine)
17. Cytovene (ganciclovir)
18. Cytovene (ganciclovir) and Zovirax (acyclovir)
19. Vitrasert (ganciclovir) intravitreal implant
20. Combivir (zidovudine/lamivudine)
21. Fuzeon (enfuvirtide)
22. Kaletra (lopinivir/ritonavir)
23. The intravenous acyclovir should be stored at room temperature.
24. Vitrasert (gancyclovir) (ocular implant)
25. NRTI, NNRTI, PI and fusion inhibitor
26. Mycostatin (nystatin)
27. Vitrasert
28. Crixivan (indinavir)
29. In order to decrease the pill load and improve compliance.
30. didanosine, zidovudine, zalcitabine

Putting Safety First

31. 250 mg once daily
32. Loading dose is 200 mg
33. 100 mg dose
34. Correct
35. 2 inhalations once daily

Understanding Concepts

36. NRTI, PI, NNRTI, and fusion inhibitors
37. Acetaminophen and/or an antihistamine
38. Itraconazole (Sporonox)
39. Kaletra
40. To prevent/treat vaginitis
41. Lozenge, clotrimazole (Mycelex)
42. NRTI (charts)
43. Post Exposure Prophylaxis
44. 1. Do not share injection equipment 2. Do not share personal items 3. Never have sex without protection
45. Nevirapine (Viramune)
46. NNRTI, nRTI, NtRTI, lactic acidosis
47. abacavir-lamivudine (Epzicom), abacavir-lamivudine-zidovudine (Trizvir), didanosine (Videx), efavirenz-emtricitabine-tenofovir (Atripla), emtricitabine (Emtriva), ganciclovir (Vitrasert), ketoconazole (Nizoral), lamivudine (Epivir), lamivudine-zidovudine (Combivir), maraviroc (Selzentry), nevirapine (Viramune), rilpivirine-tenofovir-emtricitabine (Complera), ritonavir (Norvir), tenofovir (Viread), tipranavir (aptivus), valacyclovir (Valtrex), zidovudine (Retrovir)
48. None

Matching–Terms and Definitions

49. a
50. b
51. h
52. i
53. j
54. c
55. f
56. g
57. d
58. e

Matching–Antiviral and Antifungal Drugs

59. f
60. f
61. v
62. v
63. v
64. v
65. v
66. f
67. f
68. f
69. f
70. v
71. f

Chapter 6 Anesthetics and Narcotics

Reading Drug Labels and Medication Orders

1. a. No, the total amount of acetaminophen would exceed the safe limit of 4000 mg/ 24 hours.
   b. 6000 mg or 6 g
2. pain
3. A patient-controlled analgesia (PCA) pump is a means of pain control whereby the patient can regulate, within certain limits, the administration of pain medication.
4. morphine
5. an area of the brain on which narcotics act, which in turn stimulate the vomiting center
6. prophylactic and abortive
7. in a stepwise fashion: first acetaminophen, then NSAIDS and then opioids
8. Prescribers unknowingly can overdose a patient on these drugs which can be fatal over time.
9. Neuromuscular blocking agents paralyze the patient during surgery.
10. if migraines occur more than twice a month
11. thorazine

Understanding the Larger Medical Context

12. glutamate
13. Desflurane can cause mild to severe upper respiratory tract irritation in children.
14. 30 mg, oral
15. amides
16. No, ketamine is not appropriate, because it can increase blood pressure and heart rate.

17. The autonomic nervous system regulates systems under involuntary control.
18. prodrome, aura, headache, headache relief, and postdrome
19. triptans-selective 5-HT receptor agonists
20. injection, oral liquid, and tablet
21. Flumazenil is used to reverse benzodiazepine overdose. Possible side effects include headache, nausea, vomiting, and agitation.

Dispensing and Storing Drugs

22. pharmacist
23. CIIs
24. The FDA has decided that they may be E-scribed, but some states are not in agreement and the technician will have to abide by the state law in this situation.
25. form 222
26. Count backs require counting the drugs remaining in the bottle after the prescription is dispensed.

Putting Safety First

27. lidocaine
28. 6 months or 5 refills, whichever comes first
29. 5
30. None
31. To combat escalating drug abuse

Understanding Concepts

32. Acetylcholine
33. Acetylcholine
34. Ergotamine
35. General
36. ICU
37. Addiction
38. Chemoreceptor trigger zone (CTZ)
39. aura
40. Migraine
41. CNS
42. A. CII, B. CIII, C. CII , D. CII , E. CIV

Matching–Brand and Generic Drug Names

43. g
44. h
45. e
46. a
47. f
48. d
49. b
50. c

Matching–Terms and Definitions

51. b
52. e
53. f
54. k
55. j
56. p
57. l
58. m
59. o
60. g
61. c
62. q
63. h
64. i
65. n
66. a
67. d

Chapter 7 Psychiatric and Related Drugs

Reading Drug Labels and Medication Orders

1. a. 500 mg/day × 1 tablet/250 mg = 2 tablets/day
   b. 2 tablets × 10 days = 20 tablets
2. a. 30 mg/dose × 5 mL/10 mg = 15 mL (or 1 tbsp)
   b. 240 mL/bottle × day/15 mL = 16 days

Understanding the Larger Medical Context

3. cardiotoxicity
4. tardive dyskinesia
5. Clozapine can cause a drop in white blood cell count. Counts should be obtained weekly for the duration of therapy. Weekly blood draws decreases patient compliance.

6. a. cost, b. limited adverse effects c. patient's response history
7. bupropion
8. vitamin deficiency, fatty liver tissue buildup (cirrhosis), brain damage, and dementia
9. used in treatment of Parkinson's disease
10. amobarbital (Amytal), secobarbital (Seconal)

Dispensing and Storing Drugs

11. antihistamines
12. alcohol
13. involuntary movements of the mouth, lips, and tongue
14. Celexa (citalopram)
15. Paxil (paroxetine)
16. Xanax (alprazolam)
17. antidepressants
18. doxepin
19. not a controlled substance
20. C-II
21. C-IV
22. not a controlled substance
23. C-IV
24. C-IV
25. C-IV
26. not a controlled substance
27. not a controlled substance
28. not a controlled substance

Putting Safety First

29. priapism
30. no: too many refills
31. no: must have DEA
32. no: patient added Lortab

Understanding Concepts

33. Saphris (arsenapine)
34. lithium
35. nefazodone
36. dextromethorphan/quinidine (Nuedexta)
37. a. acknowledge problem
    b. limit time spent with users
    c. seek professional help
    d. seek support from recovering alcoholic
38. Imipramine (Tofranil)
39. Budepion (Zyban)
40. Ramelton (Rozerem)
41. Haldol
42. Ramelton (Rozerem)
43. Lithium
44. Quetiapine
45. Restoril
46. Venlafaxine (Effexor)
47. Schizophrenia
48. There is no advantage.
49. Panic disorder
50. Tardive
51. Anxiety
52. OROS
53. Anorexia
54. Bipolar Disorder
55. Insomnia
56. PTSD (post traumatic stress disorder)
57. SAD (seasonal affective disorder)

Matching–Brand and Generic Drug Names

58. p
59. o
60. c
61. d
62. n
63. g
64. h
65. i
66. b
67. q
68. l
69. k
70. j
71. m
72. e
73. f
74. a

Matching–Terms and Definitions

75. b
76. a
77. h
78. i
79. e

80. c
81. d
82. g
83. f

Chapter 8 Drugs for Central Nervous System Disorders

Reading Drug Labels and Medication Orders

1. The controlled substance clonazepam cannot have more than five refills.
2. The drug is available in 50 mg tablets, so 1 tablet = 1 dose. The patient is to take 2 tablets per day (bid) for 2 days (2 tablets/day × 2 days = 4 tablets), and then 4 tablets per day (qid) for 8 days (4 tablets/day × 8 days = 32 tablets). The total tablets taken during the regimen is 4 tablets + 32 tablets = 36 tablets.
3. a. 88 kg × 1.75 mg/kg/day = 154 mg/day
   b. Yes, Imuran IV is the correct drug.
   c. 154 mg/day × 6 days = 924 mg

Understanding the Larger Medical Context

4. tonic-clonic, absence, myoclonic, atonic
5. substantia nigra
6. The addition of carbidopa reduces the amount of levodopa that is metabolized in the body. More levodopa per dose reaches the brain, allowing for less levodopa needed per dose, and fewer side effects.
7. The most common reason for failure is that the inappropriate agent is selected.
8. Diazepam (Valium) is the drug of choice followed by phenytoin or barbiturates. All are given intravenously for staticus epilepticus.
9. weakness, lacking strength in skeletal muscles, ptosis (drooping eyelids), diplopia (double vision), dysarthria (difficulty articulating), dysphagia (difficulty swallowing), respiratory difficulty
10. Lyrica (pregabalin), Cymbalta (duloxetine), Savella (milnacipran)

Dispensing and Storing Drugs

11. refrigerator
12. The bottle should be kept upside-down.
13. in a safe
14. in the refrigerator
15. antiepileptics
16. take at bedtime
17. shelf
18. antidepressants
19. guanfacine
20. baclofen (Lioresal), clobazam (Onfi), clonazepam (Klonopin), dextroamphetamine-amphetamine (Adderall), divalproex (Depakote), ethosuximide (Zarontin), gabapentin (Horizant, Neurontin), interferon beta 1a (Avenox, Rebif), interferon beta 1b (Betaseron, Extavia), lamotrigine (Lamictal), levetiracetam (Keppra), lisdexamfetamine (Vyvanse), methylphenidate (Concerta, Daytrana, Metadate ER, Methyline, Ritalin, Ritalin-SR), mitoxantrone (Novantrone), oxcarbazepine (Trileptal), phenytoin (Dilantin), pregabalin (Lyrica), primidone (Mysoline), topiramate (Topamax), valproic acid (Depakene), zonisamide (Zonegran)
21. C-IV
22. C-II
23. C-II
24. C-IV
25. C-II
26. C-IV
27. C-II
28. C-IV
29. C-V

Putting Safety First

30. Once daily
31. Should not exceed 300 mg per day
32. This is correct.
33. Once per day
34. This is correct.

Understanding Concepts

35. Crush #60 of the 400 mg tablets, mix with 600 mL of Ora Sweet. The sig will read: Take two teaspoonsful twice daily.
36. Enlon (edrophonium)

37. Valproic
38. Stalevo
39. clonazepam
40. grand
41. Myasthenia
42. multiple sclerosis
43. ptosis
44. medulla
45. Restless
46. fibromyalgia
47. status
48. partial
49. epilepsy
50. clonidine
51. selegiline (Eldepryl)
52. Strattera (atomoxetine) Catapres (clonidine) Intuniv (guanfacine)
53. Sinemet (carbidopa/levodopa)
54. Lyrica (pregabalin)

Matching–Brand and Generic Drug Names

55. g
56. d
57. a
58. c
59. f
60. e
61. b

Matching–Terms and Definitions

62. d
63. a
64. b
65. c
66. g
67. e
68. i
69. m
70. n
71. f
72. j
73. l
74. k
75. h

Chapter 9 Respiratory Drugs

Reading Drug Labels and Medication Orders

1. a. Take 1 teaspoonful by mouth every 4 to 6 hours as needed for persistent cough.
   b. "May cause drowsiness" because of the codeine and "Avoid alcohol" because alcohol increases the risk of drowsiness
2. a. 1 lozenge × 6 doses/day × 30 days/month = 180 lozenges
3. a. 4 mg tablets and 5 mg tablets
   b. Because the 4 mg tablets cannot be cut in half easily, the appropriate dosage form is 5 mg tablets; a 1 month supply would be 60 tablets (2 tabs/day) × 30 days = 60 tablets.
4. a. dose = 0.6mL, amount = 6 mL
   b. dose + 1.8 mL, amount = 18 mL
5. a. 300 mg/day × 1 cap/150 mg = 2 caps/day × 30 days/month × 3 months/treatment = 180 caps/treatment
6. a. hydroxyzine
   b. capsule, injection, oral, liquid, tablet
7. a. You could use the oral solution or you could crush the tablet form.

Understanding the Larger Medical Context

8. The dose and instructions are indicative of Flonase, the nasal spray.
9. Rinse his mouth to avoid candidiasis.
10. When using the HFA MDI inhaler, the patient should breathe in slowly. When using the dry-powder MDI inhaler, the patient should breathe in quickly.
11. a. improved performance in sports and sex
    b. better smelling home, car, clothing and breath
    c. economic savings
    d. freedom from addiction
    e. healthier babies
    f. improved health
    g. improved self-esteem
    h. improved sense of taste and smell

i. no concern regarding exposing others to smoke
j. setting a good example for children and young adults

Dispensing and Storing Drugs

12. Keep in the foil package when not being used.
13. tech
14. 120, 300 mL
15. 120, 300 mL
16. spacer
17. Cayston, Azactam (aztreonam)

Putting Safety First

18. a. he may be getting infections from the dirty nebulizer. b. The nebulizer needs to be cleaned daily.
19. Glassia (alpha one proteinase inhibitor)

Understanding Concepts

20. asthma
21. nicotine
22. A mucolytic
23. PEFR (peak expiratory flow rate)
24. MDI
25. metered dose inhaler
26. albuterol
27. mometasone/formoterol
28. mirror image
29. Astepro (azelastin)

Matching–Brand and Generic Drug Names

30. e
31. f
32. b
33. g
34. d
35. h
36. c
37. i
38. j
39. a

Matching–Terms and Definitions

40. l
41. h
42. m
43. o
44. b
45. g
46. p
47. n
48. i
49. j
50. q
51. c
52. k
53. d
54. s
55. t
56. a
57. e
58. r
59. f

Unit 3 Major Classes of Pharmaceutical Products II

Chapter 10 Drugs for Gastrointestinal and Related Diseases

Reading Drug Labels and Medication Orders

1. 1 tbsp = 15 mL; 15 mL/dose × 3 doses/day = 45 mL/day; 1 pt/bottle × 473 mL/pint × 1 day/45 mL = 10 days/bottle
2. dosage form is 300 mg capsule and prescription is for 2 capsules/day so 2 capsules/day × 30 days/month = 60 capsules/month
3. a. 2 tbsp/dose × 15 mL/1 tbsp = 30 mL/dose; 10 g/15 mL × 30 mL/dose = 20 g/dose
   b. 473 mL/bottle × 1 dose/30 mL = 15.766 dose/bottle or 15 full doses
   c. 24 hours/day × 1 dose/6 hours = 4 doses/day; 15 full doses × 1 day/4 doses = 3.75 days
4. a. Asacol 400 mg tablets
   b. Take 2 tablets by mouth three times a day.
5. bismuth subsalicylate
6. a. 2 doses/day × 600 mg/dose × 1 tablet/200 mg = 6 tablets/day
7. 150 mg/dose × 1 mL/25 mg = 6 mL/dose

Understanding the Larger Medical Context

8. Yes, the patient's BMI is 27.5. Xenical patients must have a BMI of at least 27.
9. Peginterferon alfa-2a (Pegasys) should accompany Copegus. Pegasys inhibits the replication of RNA and DNA in the virus.
10. psyllium
11. docusate (Colace)
12. Serotonin antagonists
13. Any two of the following: dolasetron (Anzemet), ganisetron (Kytril), ondansetron (Zofran)
14. A female must be tested before, every month while taking, and 6 months following if prescribed Victrelis (bocepivir).

Dispensing and Storing Drugs

15. The technician will have to prepare the drug.
16. Dexadrin (dextroamphetamine) and Desoxyn (methamphetamine)
17. Alli (orlistat)
18. It must be wiped clean to prevent cross contamination
19. Motofen (atropine/difenoxin) Lomotil (atropine/diphenoxylate)

Putting Safety First

20. The prescriber intended for the patient to take the drug two days before the trip, during the trip, and for seven days after the trip. Call MD and make sure, then make sure the pharmacist counsels patient.
21. difenoxinatropine (Motofen), diphenoxylate-atropine (Lomotil)
22. loperamide (Imodium)
23. Carafate is dosed every 6 hours.
24. Rowasa is given as a rectal enema.
25. The dose is correct.
26. A BMI of at least 30 is required to initiate treatment with Xenical.
27. Malarone should be taken 1 to 2 days before entering the malaria area.

Understanding Concepts

28. protonix (pantoprazole)
29. milk of magnesia
30. Xenical (orlistat)
31. Prevpak
32. sucralfate (Carafate)
33. quinine
34. a. Anzemet (olansetron)
    b. Kytril (grnaisetron)
    c. Zofran (ondansetron)
    d. Aloxi (palonosetron)
35. Fleet, Visicol

36. Prilosec (omeprazole)
37. Adalimumab (Humira)
38. Body Mass Index (BMI)
39. ulcer
40. Nitazoxanide (Alinia)
41. Maalox
42. adipex (phenteramine)
43. gastrointestinal
44. olsalazine (Dipentum)
45. thiabendazole (Mintezol)
46. IVIG
47. GERD (gastroesophageal reflux disease)

Matching–Brand and Generic Drug Names

48. b
49. a
50. d
51. c
52. h
53. g
54. i
55. k
56. j
57. f
58. e

Matching–Terms and Definitions

59. d
60. f
61. j
62. q
63. e
64. i
65. a
66. o
67. g
68. l
69. b
70. c
71. m
72. k
73. h
74. n
75. p

Chapter 11 Renal System Drugs

Reading Drug Labels and Medication Orders

1. a. 420 mL
   b. 33 days
2. a. tablet
   b. 90
   c. two
   d. shelf at room temperature
3. a. by injection
   b. 3 months
4 a. 80 days
5. a. The 2 mL size should be used because it will not cause any waste.

Understanding the Larger Medical Context

6. *E. coli*
7. hyperkalemia (high serum potassium levels), gynecomastia
8. loss of reserve, insufficient, chronic insufficiency, and end-stage renal disease
9. filtration, absorption and excretion
10. fatigue, heat and cold intolerance, altered tastes, loss of appetite, and anemia are detectable to the patient. Lab tests will show hyperphosphatemia, hypocalcemia, hyperkalemia, and uremia. Creatinine clearance will be low.

Dispensing and Storing Drugs

11. Osmitol (mannitol)
12. D_5W
13. MG
14. MG
15. N
16. N
17. N
18. N
19. N
20. N
21. B
22. MG
23. N

24. Nephrocaps has folic acid and other B vitamins, and vitamin C.
25. radiocontrast dyes
26. sucralfate, aluminum-containing antacids
27. pentosan polysulfate sodium (Elmiron)
28. methenamine (Cystex, Hiprex, Urex)
29. tamsulosin (Flomax)
30. oxybutynin (Ditropan, Oxytrol) and tolterodine (Detrol)
31. a. osmotic diuretics
    b. thiazide diuretics
    c. loop diuretics
    d. carbonic anhydrase inhibitors

Putting Safety First

32. Furosemide increases potassium secretion
33. Any of these three: anticholinergics, oral bronchodilators, TCAs (tricyclic antidepressants), calcium channel blockers, disopyramide, antihistamines
34. Hydrochlorothiazide
35. Prevents wasting potassium
36. Dyazide, Maxzide
37. Alpha-1 blockers
38. Eplerenone (Inspra)
39. Overactive bladder
40. Phenazopyridine (Azo Standard, Uristat)
41. Duloxetine (Cymbalta)
42. BPH
43. Nocturia
44. Nephron
45. Filtration
46. ESRD

Matching–Brand and Generic Drug Names

47. i
48. e
49. g
50. d
51. a
52. h
53. b
54. f
55. c

Matching–Terms and Definitions

56. a
57. f
58. i
59. d
60. j
61. c
62. e
63. h
64. b
65. g

Chapter 12 Drugs for Cardiovascular Diseases

Reading Drug Labels and Medication Orders

1. a. 4 patches; 1 patch/week × 4 weeks/month = 4 patches
   b. 4 patches and 4 pieces of adhesive overlay to hold the patch with the active ingredient
2. a. 4 g/dose × 3 doses/day = 12 g/day
   b. contents of one package to be mixed with 4 to 6 fl oz of liquid
3. a. 18 mL
4. a. Toprol-XL
5. a. losartan and hydrochlorothiazide
   b. 12.5 mg day × 30 days/month = 375 mg/month
6. a. Since the patient could receive a maximum of 4 vials/day, 4 vials/day × 5 days = 20 vials.
7. a. Lovenox 100 mg/mL syringes
   b. (90 mg dose) × (1 mL/100 mg) = 0.9 mL
8. a. enteric coated
   b. Baby aspirin comes in doses of 81 mg, or about one-fourth of the adult dose.
9. a. 125 mg/(100 mL NS + 25 mL drug) = 1 mg/mL
   b. in the refrigerator

Understanding the Larger Medical Context

10. An ACEI (angiotensin-converting enzyme) inhibitors work by blocking angiotensin-converting enzymes to prevent the conversion of antiotensin I to antiotensin II, a potent vasoconstrictor. An ARB (angiotensin H receptor blocker) binds to the angiotensin II receptors, thereby blocking the vasoconstriction effects of these receptors.
11. isorbide-hydralazine (BiDil), African American population
12. to reduce dizziness
13. Total < 200, LDL <100, HDL > 60, triglycerides <50
14. Nebivelol (Bystolic) causes vasodilation by increasing the production of nitric acid.
15. HDL
16. LDL
17. The manufacturer fixes the doses. However, prescribers sometimes use a dose based on body weight. In these latter cases, the person who administers the drug uses only part of the contents of a syringe and disposes of the rest of the drug. If a pharmacy technician receives a prescription for a fraction of a dose, or of a mixed dose, check with the prescriber to ensure accuracy.
18. The correct aspirin is 325 mg, uncoated. An enteric coated aspirin would take too long to get into the blood stream
19. to decrease pill load and improve patient compliance

Dispensing and Storing Drugs

20. yes
21. yes
22. no
23. yes
24. no
25. yes
26. yes
27. no
28. yes
29. no
30. no
31. no (only brand Procardia)
32. yes
33. no
34. no
35. bbw
36. n
37. b
38. b
39. b
40. n
41. n
42. n
43. mg
44. mg
45. n
46. n
47. bbw
48. b
49. n
50. bbw
51. n
52. mg
53. n
54. n

Putting Safety First

55. Coumadin (warfarin), Pradaxa (dabigatran), Xarelto (rivaroxaban)
56. Loniten (minoxidil), Nitropress (nitroprusside)
57. Trilipix (fenofibric acid)
58. no: comes in 25, 50, and 100 mg
59. no: given in two injections of 10 mLs

Understanding Concepts

60. 7 days
61. Retavase (reteplase)
62. Dilantin (phenytoin)
63. heparin
64. angina
65. cholesterol
66. MI
67. triglycerides
68. Congestive heart failure
69. arrhythmia
70. bradycardia

71. diastolic
72. thrombosis
73. Viagra (sildenafil)
74. reduced bleeding
    reliable dose response
    longer plasma half-life
    no effect on platelets
    no need for monitoring
    manufactured in syringe with needles attached

Matching–Drug Names and Drug Groups

75. cc
76. f
77. v
78. p
79. z
80. a
81. t
82. u
83. i
84. h
85. x
86. g
87. s
88. ee
89. d
90. c
91. k
92. q
93. aa
94. e
95. m
96. y
97. r
98. b
99. l
100. dd
101. ff
102. w
103. bb
104. n
105. o
106. j

Matching–Terms and Definitions

107. w
108. f
109. g
110. o
111. b
112. l
113. c
114. j
115. d
116. m
117. t
118. r
119. q
120. i
121. u
122. a
123. h
124. k
125. n
126. v
127. s
128. p
129. e
130. x

Chapter 13 Drugs for Muscle and Joint Disease and Pain

Reading Drug Labels and Medication Orders

1. a. Yes, all NSAIDs require a Medication Guide when dispensed.
   b. Take with food.
2. a. disease-modifying antirheumatic drug (DMARD)
   b. Enbrel is indicated in the treatment of moderate to severe rheumatoid arthritis in patients who have experienced an inadequate response to one or more of the other arthritis drugs.
3. a. OTC
   b. 3.2 g/day
4. 4 grams per day

5. No too much acetaminophen, more than 4 grams

Understanding the Larger Medical Context

6. A muscle is an organ that produces movement by contracting. A joint is a place of union or junction between two or more bones
7. Prevent addictions
8. The side effects of muscle relaxants are sedation, reduced mental alertness, reduced motor abilities, and GI upset.
9. Unlike osteoarthritis which affects cartilage, rheumatoid arthritis is characterized by inflammation of the joint's synovial membrane. Osteoarthritis is a degenerative joint disease resulting in loss of cartilage, elasticity, and thickness. Rheumatoid arthritis is an autoimmune disease in which the body's immune system attacks its own connective tissue.
10. COX-1 and COX-2 are enzymes that speed the production of prostaglandins that cause inflammation and pain. COX-1 is found at the site of inflammation as well as the stomach, while COX-2 is found at the site of inflammation, but not in the stomach.
11. NSAIDs work by inhibiting prostaglandin synthesis in tissue, preventing pain receptor sensitization and inflammation.
12. The combination of an opiate, which works to reduce pain centrally, and an NSAID, which works at the site of pain, allows for a lowered dose of narcotic. The lower dose facilitates the treatment of pain and reduces the risk of dependency.
13. DMARDs act to slow the progression of rheumatoid arthritis and they can prevent joint damage from occurring. DMARDs are limited by side effects. The most common side effects are immunosuppression and liver damage.
14. Gout is a disease resulting from the overproduction or improper excretion of uric acid by the body. The extra uric acid crystallizes and precipitates. The sharp crystals make their way into joints (affecting the feet and toes first) and cause great pain.
15. stomach ulceration. It can be minimized by taking with food.
16. drug containing both a narcotic and an NSAID
17. acetylcysteine
18. tramadol (Ultram)
19. celexicob (Celebrex)
20. Any of the five tips: take with food, use antacids, do not use gastric irritants such as alcohol, stop the NSAID before any elective surgical procedure (7 days with aspirin, 1 to 2 days with other NSAIDs), use the lowest possible dose, be aware of side effects, take sufficient fluids, if sensitive to aspirin avoid NSAIDS, use the lowest possible dose
21. indomethicin and ketorlac
22. naproxen and ibuprofen

Dispensing and Storing Drugs

23. Take with food.
24. no
25. NSAIDS
26. Dantrium (dantrolene)
27. NSAIDS

Putting Safety First

28. Colcrys (colchicine) Indocin (indomethacin) Krystexxa (pegloticase)
29. acetaminophen
30. 4 grams
31. Liver damage can occur at this dose

Understanding Concepts

32. Remicade (infliximab)
33. Indocin (indomethacin)
34. Valium (diazepam)
35. Aleve (naproxen)
36. Tylenol (acetaminophen)
37. gout
38. diclofenac
39. ibuprofen
40. Celebrex (celecoxib)
41. Ultracet
42. Motrin, Advil
43. hypotension
44. hypertension
45. Ultram

46. Acetylcholine
47. DMARDS
48. rheumatoid
49. Rye's
50. NSAIDS
51. visceral
52. gout
53. somatic
54. arthritis
55. spasticity
56. gouty

Matching–Drug Names and Drug Groups

57. h
58. k
59. g
60. b
61. c
62. j
63. i
64. e
65. d
66. f
67. a

Matching–Terms and Definitions

68. n
69. j
70. p
71. l
72. o
73. k
74. r
75. h
76. i
77. e
78. f
79. d
80. g
81. m
82. b
83. c
84. a
85. q

Chapter 14 Hormonal Disorders and Their Treatment

Reading Drug Labels and Medication Orders

1. a. The pills are in blister packs that tell the patient exactly how to take the drugs. All the information would not fit on a label. Day 1: 2 tablets before breakfast, one after lunch, one after supper, two before bed; Day 2: 1 tablet before breakfast, one after lunch, one after supper, two before bed; Day 3: 1 tablet before breakfast, one after lunch, one after supper, one before bed; Day 4: 1 tablet before breakfast, one after lunch, one before bed; Day 5: 1 tablet before breakfast and one before bed; Day 6: 1 tablet before breakfast
2. DAW means dispense as written. Prescribers write DAW because the small difference allowed by the FDA for generic drugs could affect the labs of a patient.
3. a. No, Glucotrol XL is an extended-release product that is only dosed once daily. You need generic glipizide or regular-release Glucotrol to properly fill this prescription.
   b. Glucotrol is in the sulfonylurea class of drugs and stimulates the pancreas to release insulin.
   c. The patient should monitor glucose levels because Glucotrol can easily cause hypoglycemia, characterized by dizziness, nausea, and headache.
4. a. 44 kg × 0.35 mg/kg/week = 15.4 mg/week
   b. 15.4 mg/week × 1 week/7 days = 2.2 mg/day
   c. 2.2 mg/day × 1 mL/4 mg = 0.55 mL/day
   d. After reconstitution, Humatrope cartridges are stable for 28 days when refrigerated. Avoid freezing.

Understanding the Larger Medical Context

5. Taking a beta blocker may interfere with the signs and symptoms of hypoglycemia. As a result, a hypoglycemic episode could go unnoticed until too late for treatment. Beta blockers can also interfere with glucose metabolism, causing hyperglycemia. Five of the following: confusion, double vision, headache, hunger, nervousness, numbness and tingling in mouth and lips, palpitations, sweating, thirst, visual disturbances, and weakness
6. People with type I diabetes cannot produce their own insulin. Type I diabetes occurs most commonly in children and young adults, but it may occur at any age. Type II diabetes is characterized by insulin insufficiency or by the resistance of the target tissues to the insulin produced. Gestational diabetes occurs during pregnancy and increases the risk of fetal morbidity and death. The onset occurs during the second and third trimesters. Secondary diabetes occurs due to certain drug use. Secondary diabetes may return to normal when the drug is discontinued.
7. Cretinism arises in children as a result of congenital (at birth) hypothyroidism, often caused by an iodine deficiency in the mother's diet during pregnancy. Cretinism can cause severe mental retardation and is marked by a thick tongue, lethargy, lack of response to commands, and short stature.
8. Non-medication causes of impotence can be low levels of testosterone, alcoholism, tobacco use, and psychological factors.
9. Menopause begins when a woman has not menstruated for one year, due to the declining rate of estrogen production. During menopause, women may experience hot flashes, vaginal dryness and atrophy, insomnia, and mood changes. Depression may also be related to menopause.
10. A false-negative can be produced from chilled or diluted urine, from medications used to treat pancreatic enzymatic insufficiency, or from testing too soon after conception. A false-positive can be produced from faulty urine collecting methods, a recent abortion, or elevated levels of human chorionic gonadotropin (HCG) due to a tumor.
11. Osteoclasts are cells that are found in the bone. They reabsorb old bone so that new bone may be formed. Osteoblasts are cells that make new bone.
12. The main reason for using corticosteroids is to inhibit inflammation. Corticosteroids are used to treat asthma, rashes, and skin disorders.
13. Insulin is a protein, and, as a protein, it would be denatured by gastric acid as soon as it reached the stomach.
14. Patients with hyperthyroidism experience decreased menses, diarrhea, flushing of the skin, heat intolerance, nervousness, increased perspiration, tachycardia, and weight loss. Adults with hyperthyroidism may have heart problems.

Dispensing and Storing Drugs

15. in the refrigerator
16. in the refrigerator
17. in the refrigerator
18. normal inventory
19. in the refrigerator
20. yes
21. no
22. yes
23. no
24. The combination of estrogen and nicotine can cause blood to clot.
25. Testosterone substances are classified as Schedule III.
26. dispense as written - may not use any other drug, even generic
27. The pharmacist needs to explain that on the first day, no matter what time the patient starts taking the drug, the whole first row is taken. The technician cannot counsel the patient.

Putting Safety First

28. testosterone
29. Flagyl (metronidazole)
30. 28 days

31. once a week
32. A dose of Zometa should not exceed 4 mg and should not be administered in less than 15 minutes.

Understanding Concepts

33. metformin
34. Regranex
35. risedronate
36. humalog
37. Striant
38. Cialis (tadalafil)
39. Viagra (silendafil)
40. authorized
41. Premarin
42. Glucovance
43. vitamin D
44. antibiotic
45. Yaz
46. osteoblast
47. thyroid
48. tricycling
49. PID
50. four
51. a) less pain; b) less PMS; c) fewer headaches; d) less endometriosis
52. Ease symptoms of menopause and strengthen bones

Matching–Drug Names and Drug Groups

53. f
54. m
55. q
56. e
57. c
58. l
59. k
60. b
61. g
62. j
63. i
64. h
65. o
66. n
67. a
68. p
69. d

Matching–Terms and Definitions

70. h
71. g
72. i
73. d
74. c
75. f
76. e
77. a
78. j
79. l
80. b
81. k

Chapter 15 Topical, Ophthalmic, and Otic Medications

Reading Drug Labels and Medication Orders

1. a. No, the prescription is written for Renova cream, which is the same drug, but in a moisturizing base. These products are not interchangeable.
   b. It makes the top layer of skin less adherent to the bottom layers, allowing it to come off more easily and quickly than with normal skin renewal. The new layer of skin underneath is smoother and wrinkle free.
2. No, for multiple lesions of impetigo, systemic therapy with an antibiotic is recommended. A localized lesion can be treated with mupirocin (Bactroban) cream or ointment. The pharmacy technician should notify the prescriber or the pharmacist.
3. The patient positions his or her head so that no liquid will drain out of the ear canal. The ear canal is filled with Cerumenex and plugged with a cotton ball. The wax softener should sit for 15 minutes, and then the ear is flushed with water.

Understanding the Larger Medical Context

4. Creams and ointments are not interchangeable. Substituting a cream for an ointment on a dermatologist's prescription could produce a failed treatment. In general, a dry skin problem is treated with an ointment, and a wet skin problem is treated with a cream.
5. Acne is an inflammation of the skin, usually on the face and neck, that is caused by increased activity of the sebaceous glands.
6. The physician may prescribe an ophthalmic agent to be used in the ear. Prescribing an ophthalmic agent for the ear is common and effective practice. However, an otic agent that is put in the eyes is very painful.
7. Open-angle glaucoma occurs when the drainage canals become clogged over time, and intraocular pressure slowly and gradually increases. It is not painful and can be treated with medication. Narrow-angle glaucoma occurs when the drainage canals become blocked. Intraocular pressure rises dramatically, and can be very painful. Medication does not treat this form, so surgery is necessary. Open-angle glaucoma is more common.
8. As a technician, be sure to put auxiliary labels on prescription products that can increase sun sensitivity. You should be familiar with all products that can increase sun sensitivity and can counsel patients on the benefits of sunscreen to help prevent sunburn and lower the risk of skin cancer.
9. UV-A and UV-B are different spectrums of light that affect human skin. A sunscreen must protect against both UV-A and UV-B rays and should contain a combination of oxybenzone and para-aminobenzoic acid or combinations of other agents that block both UV-A and UV-B rays. Avobenzone, titanium dioxide, or zinc oxide protect against dangerous UV wavelengths. Sunscreen should contain a rating of at least SPF (sunburn protection factor) of 15.
10. Pull down on the lower eyelid, apply a small ribbon of ointment, and then let go of the eyelid. Blink a few times to spread the ointment. Becausue vision may be blurry for a few minutes, do only one eye at a time.
11. The patient should wait at least 5 minutes between applications.
12. The OTC medications may be as effective as the prescription drugs for treating head lice and may cause fewer side effects.

Dispensing and Storing Drugs

13. n
14. n
15. n
16. n
17. n
18. n
19. b
20. n
21. n
22. n

Putting Safety First

23. head lice
24. The indication is correct.
25. acne
26. The indication is correct.
27. The indication is correct.
28. ear wax removal
29. The indication is correct.
30. genital warts or psoriasis
31. female facial hair removal
32. The indication is correct.

Understanding Concepts

33. Hibiclens (chlorhexadine)
34. Vaniqa (eflornithing)
35. Natacyn (natamycin)
36. Solage (mequinol/tretoin)
37. psoriasis
38. acne
39. candidiasis
40. dermis
41. humor
42. keratosis
43. glaucoma
44. epidermis
45. dermatitis

46. melanoma
47. atopic
48. photosensitivity
49. conjunctivitis
50. teratogenic
51. wart
52. SPF

Matching–Brand and Generic Drug Names

53. c
54. a
55. d
56. b
57. i
58. f
59. j
60. g
61. h
62. e

Matching–Terms and Definitions

63. g
64. a
65. c
66. b
67. e
68. f
69. d

Unit 4 Chemotherapy and Miscellaneous Pharmaceutical Products

Chapter 16 Recombinant Drugs and Chemotherapy

Reading Drug Labels and Medication Orders

1. a. BSA = 2.15 m^2
   b. 400 mg/m^2 × 2.15 m^2 = 860 mg, 860 mg × 1 mL/50 mg = 17.2 mL
   c. D_5W, 250 mL
   d. 85 mg/m^2 × 2.15 m^2 = 182.75 mg; 182.75 mg/dose × 1 vial/50 mg = 3.655 vials/dose, round to 4 vials/dose; 4 vials/dose × 3 cycles = 12 vials/3 cycles
   e. 3 mL/hour × 46 hours = 138 mL
2. a. 400 mg/m^2 × 2.15 m^2 = 860 mg
   b. 860 mg/dose × 1 vial/100 mg = 8.6 vials/dose, rounded to 9 vials
3. a. 40,000 units × 1 mL/10,000 units = 4 mL
   b. 40,000 units/dose × 1 vial/20,000 units = 2 vials
4. a. 20 mg/day × 30 days/month = 600 mg/month
   b. Take 2 tablets by mouth daily.
5. Since 25 mg/5 mL per drug label: 65 mg × 5 mL/25 mg = 13 mL.
6. 60 mL of each ingredient
7. a. BSA = 1.80 m^2
   b. 175 mg/m^2 × 1.80 m^2 = 315 mg; 315 mg/dose × 1 mL/6mg = 52.5 mL
   c. 500 mg/dose × 10 mg/mL = 50 mL/dose

Understanding the Larger Medical Context

8. Immunosuppression is the inhibition of the immune system by which the body fights infections. Immunosuppression is a deliberate therapy in transplant patients to prevent the immune system from rejecting the transplanted organ. (Immunosuppression is also a consequence of some diseases, such as AIDS.) A patient who is immunosuppressed may be more susceptible to infections. Long-term immunosuppression complications include cancer, renal failure, and diabetes.
9. B-cells provide memory, or the ability to remember an antigen in the event T-cells have the ability to attack a specific antigen.

10. Type I reactions have multiple components that can be pharmacologically treated. Albuterol for sympathomimetic reactions, epinephrine for catecholamines, and corticosteroids for inflammatory responses.
11. Neupogen and Neulasta have the same parent protein (filgrastim). However, Neulasta is a pegylated form, which causes the drug to act longer to maintain sufficient white blood cell counts.

Dispensing and Storing Drugs

12. Epogen, Procrit (epogen alpha)
13. Zortress (everolimus)
    Cellcept (mycophenolate)
    Rapamune (sirolimus)
14. Tasigna (nilotinib)
    Votrient (pazopanib)
    Caprelsa (randetanib)
15. Novaldex (tamoxifen)

Putting Safety First

16. Neupogen is incompatible with normal saline and should be mixed in 5% dextrose.
17. Only 1 dose of Neulasta is given after a cycle of chemotherapy.
18. Proleukin treatment consists of two 5 day treatment cycles separated by a rest period of 9 days.
19. Mylotarg is infused over 2 hours and is good for 20 days after reconstitution.
20. To use Xeloda, a daily dose is administered in 2 divided doses, 12 hours apart.

Understanding Concepts

21. swizzle
22. Nitrogen
23. monoclonal antibody
24. Alkylating
25. Plant
26. Provenge (sipuleucel-T)
27. Halaven (eribulin)
28. biological safety
29. Gloves
30. hand

Matching–Drug Names and Drug Groups

31. e
32. c
33. d
34. f
35. a
36. b
37. i
38. g
39. j
40. h

Matching Drug with Malignancy

41. i
42. f
43. k
44. e
45. h
46. j
47. m
48. n
49. b
50. a
51. d
52. l
53. c
54. g

Matching–Terms and Definitions

55. h
56. g
57. j
58. f
59. b
60. e
61. d
62. a
63. i
64. c

Chapter 17 Vitamins, OTC Supplements, Antidotes, and Miscellaneous Topics

Reading Drug Labels and Medication Orders

1. a. Yes, this prescription is okay to fill as written.
   b. It is okay to dispense Cipro 250 mg instead. You would have to dispense 240 tablets to complete the 60 day supply.
2. a. Digibind 38 mg or Digifab 40 mg
   b. The empiric treatment is 20 vials of either Digibind or Digifab IV in two divided doses.

Understanding the Larger Medical Context

3. Calcium gluconate prevents a negative calcium balance, moderates muscle and nerve performance and allows normal cardiac function. Calcium chloride is for cardiac resuscitation when patients fail. Calcium carbonate is an antacid. Calcium acetate is used to control hyperphosphatemia and end stage renal function. Calcium citrate is used as a supplement along with vitamin D and is preferred for the elderly because it is better absorbed.
4. PN is a nutrient solution administered through a vein. TPN is an amino acid-dextrose-lipid solution used for PM.
5. They are sold as a food and have no FDA quality control, but the poison laws of the FDA apply.
6. Stabilize patient and then transport to a site of continuing care
7. vomiting, diarrhea, edema, sweat, weight loss
8. If a hypotonic solution is administered, water from the solution may enter the cells to reach equilibrium. This could cause the cells to swell. If a hypertonic solution is administered, water from the cells may shift to the extracellular space to reach equilibrium. This could cause the cells to shrink.
9. The main issues are: (1) the possibility that one herb may be mistaken for another, resulting in serious side effects or an allergic response; (2) the potential for interactions with other herbs and drugs; and (3) the possibility that a patient will initially treat a disease with herbs and forgo effective pharmaceutical treatment until the disease is too far advanced to realize the full benefits of drug therapy.
10. A pharmacy technician can document drug allergies, keep records of who receives which drugs, and maintain patient profiles.
11. Occasionally dobutamine will turn a slight pink color, but this color change does not indicate a significant loss of potency. As long as dobutamine has been properly stored, it should retain its potency until the printed expiration date. You do not need to replace the drug.

Dispensing and Storing Drugs

12. Rx
13. Rx
14. OTC
15. OTC
16. Rx
17. Rx
18. OTC
19. OTC
20. OTC
21. OTC

Putting Safety First

22. The electrolytes calcium and phosphorus are most likely to precipitate. Phosphorus should be added next, and mixed thoroughly. The calcium (acetate form) can then be added to the final product.
23. Epinephrine is used to treat emergency cardiac arrest and to help stabilize ventricular fibrillation.
24. The three types of anthrax are cutaneous, inhalation, oropharyngeal and gastrointestinal. Anthrax is treated with antibiotics.
25. Ricin is a toxin that is derived from the castor bean. Ricin disables the molecular machinery for protein synthesis.

26. Vitamins A, D, E, and K are fat-soluble. The fat-soluble vitamins are absorbed with dietary fats and are maintained in stores by the body, mainly in the liver. As excessive amounts collect, signs of toxicity develop.

Understanding Concepts

27. chamomile
28. Deplin
29. amyl
30. charcoal
31. Wort
32. Dapsone
33. Anascorp (centruroides immune F)
34. Glucerna
35. Jevity
36. Thiamine
37. D2
38. niacin
39. acidophilus
40. Nepro
41. Kava
42. Align
43. Folic
44. Ascorbic
45. antidote
46. ricin
47. osteomalacia
48. cracking
49. acidosis
50. alkalosis
51. blue

Matching–Drug Names and Drug Groups

52. a
53. b
54. d
55. c
56 e
57. g
58. j
59. h
60. i
61. f

Matching–Terms and Definitions

62. g
63. i
64. c
65. d
66. m
67. f
68. a
69. h
70. b
71. n
72. l
73. k
74. j
75. e

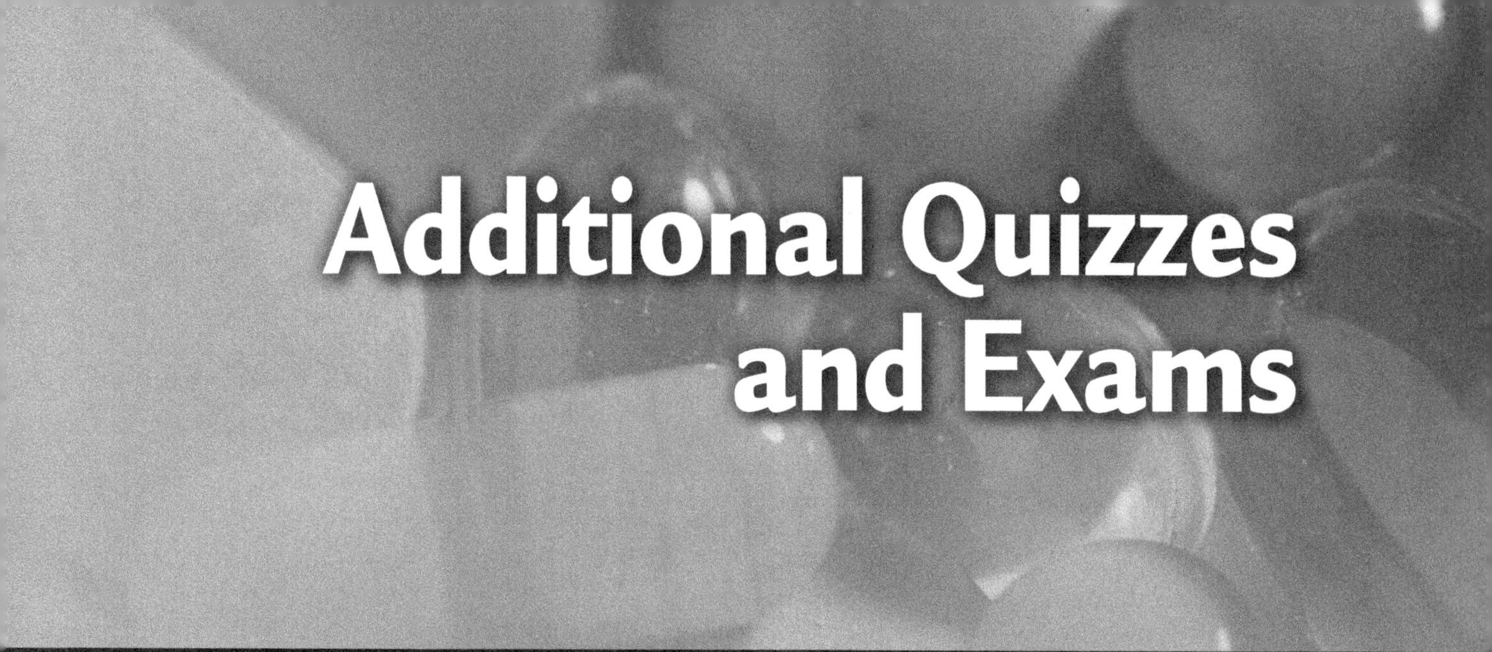

Additional Quizzes and Exams

This section includes quizzes for all 17 chapters as well as a variety of exams, including tests for each of the four units, a midterm exam that covers Units 1 and 2 and a midterm exam that covers Units 3 and 4, and a comprehensive final exam. None of these questions appear on the Study Partner CD. Electronic files for these quizzes and exams are available on the password-protected Internet Resource Center (Web site) for this title at www.paradigmcollege.net/pharmacology5e.

Answer Keys for all of these quizzes and exams appear at the end of this section.

Chapter Quizzes

Chapter 1 Evolution of Medicinal Drugs

Multiple Choice

Identify the choice that best completes the statement or answers the question.

1. What is a meaning of the root of the word for pharmacology (*pharmakon*) in the early Greek language?
   a. sleep
   b. antibiotic
   c. magic spell
   d. history
   e. antidote

2. What is an apothecary?
   a. a greenhouse for growing medicinal plants
   b. a publication listing common medical preparations available in individual hospitals or communities
   c. a science dealing with the preparation of herbal medications
   d. forerunner of today's pharmacists in England

3. During what time frame of American history did the boundaries between physician and pharmacist become clearly delineated?
   a. 1492–1535 (settling of America)
   b. 1776–1784 (American Revolution)
   c. 1861–1865 (Civil War)
   d. 1914–1918 (World War I)
   e. 1939–1945 (World War II)

4. What organization was established in 1852 to counter the encroachment of other medical areas into pharmacy?
   a. American Medical Association (AMA)
   b. American Pharmaceutical Association (APhA)
   c. Pharmaceutical Manufacturers of America (PMA)
   d. International Association of Formulators and Dispensers (IAFD)

5. What is another term for a drug's United States Adopted Name (USAN)?
   a. chemical
   b. generic
   c. trade
   d. brand

6. What did the Food, Drug and Cosmetic Act of 1938 require of new drugs before they could be marketed in the United States?
   a. safety
   b. efficacy
   c. nonaddictiveness
   d. affordability

7. What phase of clinical trials is carried out after the drug has been approved for marketing?
   a. phase I
   b. phase II
   c. phase III
   d. phase IV
   e. phase V

8. When is a drug studied in patients who have the condition that the drug is intended to treat?
   a. phase I
   b. phase II
   c. phase III
   d. phase IV

9. Drugs from which FDA Pregnancy Category can safely be used in pregnant patients?
   a. A
   b. B
   c. C
   d. D
   e. X

10. Into how many schedules are controlled substances categorized in the United States?
   a. 2
   b. 3
   c. 4
   d. 5
   e. 6

11. What is *not* true of FDA-approved generic drugs?
   a. They must contain the same active ingredients as the original drug.
   b. Although they may have a new generic name or USAN, generic drugs may keep the trade name of the original drug.
   c. Generic drugs must be identical in strength, dosage form, and route of administration to the original drug.
   d. They must have the same indications as the original drug.

12. Manufacturers of foods containing which ingredients may make health claims regarding the disease-fighting action of the food?
   a. whole grains
   b. simple carbohydrates
   c. unsaturated fats
   d. gluten
   e. low fat

13. Which group listed below is an organization of educators that focuses on pharmacy technician curriculums?
   a. PTCB
   b. PTEC
   c. AAPT
   d. APhA
   e. NABP

14. What event forced American physicians and druggists to make their own drugs?
   a. French and Indian War
   b. American Revolution
   c. War of 1812
   d. Civil War
   e. World War I

15. The first chemical agent used to treat a disease was
   a. carbolic acid.
   b. arsphenamine.
   c. insulin.
   d. prontosil.
   e. penicillin.

16. Which task might a pharmacy technician in a hospital pharmacy perform?
    a. prepare sterile IVs and chemotherapy compounds
    b. conduct a "tech check tech" in the preparation of medicine carts
    c. educate nurses about pharmacy-related issues
    d. a and c
    e. a, b, and c

17. What is the source of thyroid?
    a. plants
    b. animal products
    c. minerals
    d. synthetic materials
    e. bioengineering

18. Professionals and consumers can report serious adverse drug reactions to
    a. MedWatch.
    b. the DEA.
    c. the USP-NF.
    d. the PTCB.
    e. the NABP.

19. A Black Box warning
    a. alerts prescribers to the known problems with the use of the drug.
    b. allows the prescriber to weigh the advantage of using this drug with its risks.
    c. is on thousands of drugs on the market.
    d. a, b, and c

20. A rating system devised by the FDA to establish the therapeutic equivalent of generic drugs is the
    a. pass/fail system.
    b. +/− system.
    c. thumbs-up system.
    d. one/two system.
    e. A/B system.

Chapter 2 Basic Concepts of Pharmacology

Multiple Choice

Identify the choice that best completes the statement or answers the question.

1. What can drugs combine with in addition to receptors?
    a. enzymes
    b. transport proteins
    c. nucleic acids
    d. All of the above

2. What does the abbreviation ADME stand for?
    a. agonist, dose, mechanism, endogenous
    b. antagonist, distribution, mechanism, external
    c. absorption, drug, metabolism, endogenous
    d. absorption, distribution, metabolism, elimination

3. What form of a drug crosses cell membranes easily?
    a. nonionized
    b. ionized
    c. Both ionized and nonionized drugs cross cell membranes easily.
    d. Neither ionized nor nonionized drugs readily cross cell membranes.

4. By what process can one drug increase the metabolism of both itself and other drugs?
    a. inhibition
    b. bioavailability
    c. first-pass
    d. induction
    e. affinity

5. What term is used to describe the phenomenon in which elevating a dose of drug no longer improves the clinical effect for that drug?
    a. potency
    b. ceiling effect
    c. peak vs. trough effect
    d. first-pass
    e. clearance

6. What is the elimination process of most drugs in which a constant fraction of the drug is eliminated per unit of time?
   a. volume distribution
   b. half-life
   c. first-order
   d. zero-order

7. If a drug has a half-life of 6 hours and a starting blood concentration of 100 mg/kg, how long will it take until the concentration of the drug in blood is 25 mg/kg?
   a. 3 hours
   b. 6 hours
   c. 12 hours
   d. 24 hours

8. What term is used to describe a severe response to a chemical that is characterized by life-threatening respiratory distress and shock?
   a. allergic sensitivity
   b. anaphylactic reaction
   c. idiosyncratic reaction
   d. active immunity

9. Which statement is *not* true about receptors?
   a. Receptors are protein molecules.
   b. Receptors are located in extra-cellular fluid.
   c. There are different types of receptors throughout the body.
   d. Receptors and chemical messengers must have complementary structures to bind.
   e. Receptors play a role in blood clotting and smooth muscle contraction.

10. What statement is *true* about lipids?
    a. They are protein molecules.
    b. They generally attract water.
    c. They generally repel water.
    d. They are not part of the cell membrane.

11. Which route of administration does *not* require absorption?
    a. oral
    b. topical
    c. rectal
    d. intravenous
    e. transdermal

12. The first main phase of the pharmacokinetic process is
    a. absorption of drug into bloodstream.
    b. absorption of drug by the liver.
    c. distribution of drug to organs and tissues.
    d. metabolism of drug by the liver.

13. Which process involves bringing a drug to its sites of action?
    a. elimination
    b. absorption
    c. distribution
    d. metabolism

14. The rate at which a drug is eliminated from a specific volume of blood per unit of time is referred to as its
    a. duration of action.
    b. metabolism.
    c. clearance.
    d. distribution.

15. Some drugs may be administered by injection because they have substantial
    a. side effects.
    b. therapeutic effects.
    c. first-pass effects.
    d. ceiling effects.

16. How can the length of time required to achieve a drug's therapeutic level be shortened?
    a. accelerate the duration of action
    b. analyze a patient blood sample and adjust dosage accordingly
    c. vary doses and dosing intervals
    d. administer a loading dose

17. A drug's clearance is important for determining the
    a. loading dose.
    b. maintenance dose.
    c. ceiling effect.
    d. first-pass effect.

18. Taking more of your prescription painkillers than prescribed is an example of
    a. drug dependence.
    b. drug addiction.
    c. drug abuse.
    d. drug tolerance.
    e. drug intolerance.

19. The label "Do not take with antacids" is placed on a prescription container to warn patients of a potential
   a. drug interaction.
   b. allergic response.
   c. adverse side effect.
   d. a and b
   e. a, b, and c

20. A person on calcium for osteoporosis also needs to take vitamin D. Without vitamin D, the calcium cannot get into the bone. The relationship between calcium and vitamin D is an example of
   a. addition.
   b. antagonism.
   c. potentiation.
   d. synergism.

Chapter 3 Dispensing Medications

Multiple Choice

Identify the choice that best completes the statement or answers the question.

1. Which of the following statements is true about a prescription?
   a. Prescriptions can be written or oral directions for medication.
   b. Prescriptions are always written directions for medication.
   c. The term *prescription* is used in institutional settings for medication.
   d. Only a physician can issue a prescription for medication.

2. Which of the following data does *not* have to be on a prescription?
   a. prescriber's name
   b. instructions (signa)
   c. amount of drug to be dispensed
   d. phone number and address of patient

3. What peroral route is administrated when a rapid action is desired?
   a. conjunctival
   b. aural
   c. buccal
   d. transdermal

4. What abbreviation is used to describe drugs injected into a muscle?
   a. IV
   b. SC
   c. IM
   d. OD
   e. PO

5. Pediatric and geriatric patients often require lower doses of drugs than other patients because
   a. they have more rapid metabolism.
   b. their livers do not metabolize the medication as well.
   c. their kidney excretion is enhanced.
   d. they sleep more.

6. What physiologic change frequently occurs in aging patients?
   a. auditory - hearing loss
   b. pulmonary - chronic obstructive pulmonary disease (COPD)
   c. cardiovascular - hypertension and coronary artery disease
   d. urinary - decreased number of functioning nephrons and incontinence
   e. All of the above

7. What does the term *mortality* mean?
   a. active immunity
   b. rate of death from a particular disease
   c. rate of occurrence from a particular disease
   d. concentration of an antigen in the blood stream

8. What is the drug (or drug class) of choice to prevent allergic diseases?
   a. antihistamines
   b. epinephrine
   c. corticosteroids
   d. Drugs treat the symptoms of allergies and cannot cure allergic diseases.
   e. Daily treatment with corticosteroids has been shown to cure allergic rhinitis and allergic dermatitis.

9. Which of these instructions on a written prescription pertains to the "right dose"?
   a. PO
   b. take with food
   c. 4 mg
   d. hydromorphone
   e. # twenty (20)

10. What is a disadvantage of administering a drug by the peroral route?
    a. The drug generally takes longer to become effective.
    b. A professional healthcare worker must administer the drug.
    c. Administration can be painful and infection is possible.
    d. Drugs are always easily swallowed.
    e. It is the most expensive way to give medications.

11. Which route of administration allows a medication to enter the bloodstream directly?
    a. sublingual
    b. buccal
    c. intravenous
    d. rectal
    e. All of the above

12. The ophthalmic route applies to medications instilled in the
    a. nose.
    b. ear.
    c. eye.
    d. mouth.
    e. vagina.

13. Macular degeneration in the elderly is an example of a(n)
    a. optic change.
    b. gastrointestinal change.
    c. hormonal change.
    d. compositional body change.
    e. cardiovascular change.

14. Delay of absorption of some drugs is a frequent problem among elderly patients due, in part, to
    a. decreased vital capacity.
    b. changes in the endocrine system.
    c. reduction in the rate of gastric emptying.
    d. decreased albumin production.
    e. increased proportion of total body fat.

15. What is the most commonly used guide to drug administration in children?
    a. age
    b. height
    c. body surface area
    d. body weight

16. What type of immunity is acquired following vaccination?
    a. active immunity
    b. passive immunity
    c. immunocompetence
    d. immunoglobulin

17. What does the term *morbidity* mean?
    a. rate of death from a particular disease
    b. rate of occurrence of a diseased state or condition
    c. exposure to an inactivated part of an infectious organism
    d. concentration of an antibody in the bloodstream

18. Which immunization should children receive at birth?
    a. hepatitis B
    b. measles-mumps-rubella
    c. influenza
    d. diphtheria-tetanus-pertussis
    e. rotavirus

19. What is a critical role that technicians carry out?
    a. help ensure medication safety
    b. counsel patients on drug safety
    c. explain side effects to patients
    d. discuss medication schedules with patients

20. What patient information must pharmacy technicians handle?
    a. honoring an order to continue medication in patient transitions
    b. verifying addresses, dates of birth, and phone numbers of patients
    c. counseling patients
    d. making sure that tamper-resistant pads are used for oral prescriptions

Chapter 4 Antibiotics

Multiple Choice

Identify the choice that best completes the statement or answers the question.

1. What was the first true class of antibiotics?
    a. sulfonamides
    b. tetracyclines
    c. cephalosporins
    d. quinolones
    e. macrolides

2. What is true of a bacteriostatic antibiotic?
   a. It kills the invading organism.
   b. It is orally effective.
   c. It inhibits the growth or multiplication of bacteria.
   d. It is evenly distributed to both the host (patient) and the bacteria.
   e. It only affects gram-negative bacteria.
3. What term is used to describe antibiotic treatment that is begun before the results of the organism culture have been returned?
   a. antimicrobial
   b. empirical
   c. environmental
   d. nosocomial
   e. broad-spectrum
4. Why should the counting tray be swabbed with alcohol after dispensing sulfa or penicillin in the tablet form?
   a. to keep it disinfected
   b. to prevent cross-contamination
   c. to help maintain an accurate tablet count
   d. to prevent deterioration of the antibiotic
5. The most frequent form of bacterial resistance to antibiotics results when bacteria
   a. prevent the antibiotic from penetrating the bacterial cell wall.
   b. block antibiotic metabolism.
   c. destroy the antibiotic by bacterial enzymes.
   d. change their membranes so that the antibiotic no longer recognizes the bacteria.
6. The major side effects of aminoglycosides, such as amikacin or kanamycin, are
   a. nephrotoxicity
   b. ototoxicity
   c. a and b
   d. none of the above
   e. nausea
7. Which of the following drugs is associated with an adverse effect known as red man syndrome?
   a. amoxicillin (Amoxil, Trimox)
   b. vancomycin (Vancocin)
   c. chloramphenicol (Chloromycetin)
   d. metronidazole (Flagyl)
   e. clindamycin (Cleocin)
8. Which statement regarding linezolid (Zyvox) is *incorrect*?
   a. It can be used to treat methicillin-resistant *S. aureus* (MRSA).
   b. It can be used to treat vancomycin-resistant *E. faecium* (VRE).
   c. It is available in IV, oral liquid, and tablet dosage forms.
   d. It should be stored in clear glass containers.
   e. The IV form should not be administered simultaneously in the same line with other drugs.
9. Which of the following drugs is a monobactam?
   a. ertapenem
   b. meropenem
   c. loracarbef
   d. aztreonam
   e. doripenem
10. Why should tetracyclines never be dispensed past their expiration date?
    a. Controlled substances may never be dispensed past their expiration date.
    b. They lose 90% of their effectiveness 30 days past their expiration date.
    c. They have the potential for causing a fatal renal syndrome.
    d. The fine for doing so is prohibitive.
11. What is the mechanism of action of quinolones on bacteria?
    a. They antagonize the enzyme responsible for coiling and replicating DNA.
    b. They inhibit protein synthesis by combining with ribosomes.
    c. They bind to bacterial membranes, causing them to depolarize.
    d. They destroy components of the bacterium's DNA nucleus.
12. Which liquid antibiotic does not have to be stored in the refrigerator after it is mixed?
    a. amoxicillin
    b. cephalexin
    c. penicillin
    d. azithromycin
    e. cefprozil

13. What auxiliary label on antibiotic prescriptions might help to reduce antimicrobial resistance?
    a. Take with fluids.
    b. Avoid sun exposure.
    c. Take all of this medication.
    d. Do not drink alcoholic beverages while taking this medication.
    e. Take on an empty stomach.

14. What is a characteristic of Stevens-Johnson syndrome?
    a. jaundice
    b. redness of the skin
    c. anemia
    d. dehydration
    e. hives

15. Why might a dentist prescribe amoxicillin?
    a. to provide prophylaxis for patients requiring surgical dental procedures
    b. to sedate patients who are fearful of dental procedures
    c. to treat patients with tooth and gum infections who are allergic to sulfa drugs
    d. a and c

16. Which drug is primarily used to treat pulmonary infections?
    a. azithromycin (Zithromax, Z Pak)
    b. tetracycline (Sumycin)
    c. nitrofurantoin (Macrobid, Macrodantin)
    d. metronidazole (Flagyl)

17. Which term refers to low blood pressure?
    a. hypoglycemia
    b. hypoplasia
    c. hypotension
    d. hypotaxis
    e. hypostasis

18. Which antibiotic has been overused?
    a. vancomycin (Vancocin)
    b. metronidazole (Flagyl)
    c. clindamycin (Cleocin)
    d. pentamidine (NebuPent, Pentam)
    e. linezolid (Zyvox)

19. Which antibiotic is effective against bacteria, fungi, and protozoa?
    a. vancomycin (Vancocin)
    b. metronidazole (Flagyl)
    c. clindamycin (Cleocin)
    d. pentamidine (NebuPent, Pentam)
    e. linezolid (Zyvox)

20. Which quinolone has an ophthalmic dosage form?
    a. ciprofloxacin (Cipro)
    b. gatifloxacin (Tequin)
    c. gemifloxacin (Factive)
    d. a and b
    e. a, b, and c

Chapter 5 Therapy for Fungal and Viral Infections

Multiple Choice

Identify the choice that best completes the statement or answers the question.

1. How are fungal and human cells similar?
    a. They both contain cholesterol in their cell membranes.
    b. They both have a defined nucleus.
    c. They both have a rigid cell wall.
    d. Neither cell is eukaryotic.

2. How can antibiotics worsen fungal infections?
    a. Antibiotics increase the likelihood of developing resistant organisms.
    b. Antibiotics kill only the weakest fungi, leaving the strongest to survive and thrive.
    c. Antibiotics may kill the body's natural flora, which tend to keep fungi in check.
    d. Antibiotics can antagonize the uptake of antifungal drugs into the infecting fungi.

3. What aspect of the fungal cell wall is affected by amphotericin B?
    a. fluidity
    b. permeability
    c. thickness
    d. protein synthesis

4. Which drug or drug class listed below is *least* likely to be used to treat side effects associated with amphotericin B?
   a. penicillin
   b. antiemetics
   c. acetaminophen
   d. antihistamines

5. Patients taking which of the following drugs should *not* drive at night?
   a. amphotericin B (Abelcet)
   b. fluconazole (Diflucan)
   c. voriconazole (VFEND)
   d. ketoconazole (Nizoral)

6. What pair of viruses below are examples of latent viruses?
   a. common cold and influenza
   b. common cold and herpes
   c. herpes and influenza
   d. herpes and HIV

7. Which of the following antiviral drug is also effective in treating patients with parkinsonism?
   a. acyclovir (Zovirax)
   b. foscarnet (Foscavir)
   c. ribavirin (Capegus)
   d. amantadine (Symmetrel)

8. What class of drugs are used to treat varicella?
   a. antiretrovials
   b. pencillins
   c. antifungus agents
   d. antiviral agents

9. Which of the following drugs cannot be used to treat influenza?
   a. famciclovir (Famvir)
   b. zanamivir (Relenza)
   c. oseltamivir (Tamiflu)
   d. amantadine (Symmetrel)

10. Which of the following choices represents a class of antiretroviral drugs?
    a. nucleoside reverse transcriptase inhibitor (NRTI)
    b. non-nucleoside reverse transcriptase inhibitor (NNRTI)
    c. protease inhibitor (PI)
    d. fusion inhibitor
    e. All of the above

11. Which of the following drugs acts by preventing the HIV virus from entering immune cells?
    a. enfuvirtide (Fuzeon)
    b. valacyclovir (Valtrex)
    c. acyclovir (Zovirax)
    d. efavirenz (Sustiva)
    e. didanosine (Videx)

12. Which antifungal is most often prescribed in liquid form to swish and swallow?
    a. clotrimazole (Mycelex-7)
    b. nystatin (Mycostatin)
    c. flucytosine (Ancobon)
    d. terconazole (Terazol)

13. What is the dispensing status of caspofungin (Cancidas)?
    a. OTC
    b. Rx
    c. Rx and OTC
    d. IV
    e. IM

14. How is ganciclovir (Vitrasert) administered?
    a. PO
    b. surgically implanted
    c. rectally
    d. IV
    e. IM

15. In which of these ways is a virus different from a bacterium?
    a. A virus is much larger than a bacterium.
    b. A virus can infect a bacterium.
    c. A virus reproduces by spores.
    d. A virus has a rigid cell wall.

16. The common cold is an example of a(n)
    a. generalized viral infection.
    b. chronic viral infection.
    c. systemic viral infection.
    d. fast viral infection.
    e. acute viral infection.

17. The process of vaccination
    a. primes the body's natural defenses against a certain viral strain.
    b. prevents patients from exposure to viral infection.
    c. reduces adverse side effects of antiviral drug therapy.
    d. a and b
    e. a, b, and c

18. Which antiviral agent is an ocular implant used to treat cytomegalovirus (CMV) infections?
   a. famciclovir (Famvir)
   b. cidofovir (Vistide)
   c. ganciclovir (Vitrasert)
   d. foscarnet (Foscavir)

19. Which class of antiretrovirals is associated with a humped back, facial atrophy, and breast enlargement?
   a. nucleoside reverse transcriptase inhibitors
   b. non-nucleoside reverse transcriptase inhibitors
   c. nucleotide reverse transcriptase inhibitors
   d. protease inhibitors
   e. fusion inhibitors

20. Post-exposure prophylaxis should be administered to
   a. patients with HIV/AIDS.
   b. caregivers and family members of patients with HIV/AIDS.
   c. teachers.
   d. healthcare workers who have been exposed to needle-stick injuries.

Chapter 6 Anesthetics and Narcotics

Multiple Choice

Identify the choice that best completes the statement or answers the question.

1. What are the two divisions of the peripheral nervous system?
   a. neurons and neurotransmitters
   b. brain and spinal cord
   c. autonomic and somatic
   d. sympathetic and afferent
   e. afferent and efferent

2. The primary CNS transmitter is
   a. acetylcholine.
   b. norepinephrine.
   c. dopamine.
   d. All of the above

3. Which of the following drugs are the most used preoperative sedatives?
   a. narcotics (opioids)
   b. barbiturates
   c. benzodiazepines
   d. phenothiazines

4. Which of the following drugs can be used to reverse the effects of a narcotic?
   a. naloxone (Narcan)
   b. flumazenil (Romazicon)
   c. etomidate (Amidate)
   d. a and b

5. What class of drugs can be used to reverse the effects of nondepolarizing neuromuscular blockers?
   a. adrenergic agonists
   b. barbiturates
   c. narcotic antagonists
   d. anticholinesterases

6. What are the primary opiate receptors associated with analgesia?
   a. cholinergic, dopaminergic, adrenergic
   b. mu, delta, kappa
   c. alpha, beta, gamma
   d. D1, D2, D3

7. What class of drugs is primarily used to treat migraine headaches?
   a. beta receptor agonists
   b. antihistamines
   c. corticosteroids
   d. triptans

8. Which of the following drugs is an example of a selective 5-HT receptor agonist?
   a. metoclopramide (Reglan)
   b. propranolol (Inderal)
   c. dihydroergotamine (Migranal)
   d. sumatriptan (Imitrex)

9. To what part of the nervous system do the sense organs belong?
   a. central
   b. afferent
   c. autonomic
   d. somatic
   e. efferent

10. Which is the only neurotransmitter of the parasympathetic system?
    a. norepinephrine
    b. dopamine
    c. acetylcholine
    d. epinephrine
    e. serotonin

11. What does norepinephrine act on?
    a. receptors in smooth muscle and cardiac muscle
    b. cardiac receptors and bronchodilator adrenergic receptors
    c. smooth muscle of bronchioles and GI tract
    d. alpha and beta receptors

12. Which component of a malignant hyperthermia kit is a skeletal muscle relaxant?
    a. dantrolene
    b. procainamide
    c. furosemide
    d. glucose
    e. sodium bicarbonate, 7.5%

13. Which inhalant anesthetic cannot be used during childbirth?
    a. desflurane (Suprane)
    b. enflurane (Ethrane)
    c. halothane
    d. isoflurane (Forane)
    e. nitrous oxide

14. A pain that occurs when no pain should be felt is
    a. somatic.
    b. chronic malignant.
    c. acute.
    d. sympathetically mediated.

15. Which is a principle of modern pain management?
    a. Withhold pain medication for as long as possible so that patients do not become addicted.
    b. Treat persistent pain first with strong opioids and then with weaker opioids.
    c. Allow patients themselves to regulate the amount of pain medication they receive.
    d. Decrease the current dosage by 50% when disease progression appears to slow down.

16. Which drug is used to treat opiate addiction?
    a. methohexital (Brevital)
    b. oxycodone (OxyContin)
    c. buprenorphine (Buprenex, Subutex)
    d. lorazepam (Ativan)
    e. neostigmine (Prostigmin)

17. Migraine therapy that attempts to prevent headaches from occurring is called
    a. abortive therapy.
    b. ergotamine therapy.
    c. prophylactic therapy.
    d. triptan therapy.
    e. controlled therapy.

18. Which drug or class of drugs is a prophylactic therapy for migraine headaches?
    a. beta blockers
    b. estrogen
    c. NSAIDs
    d. a and c
    e. All of the above

19. Which of the following are classified as antiemetic agents?
    a. Thorazine
    b. Reglan
    c. Compazine
    d. a and b
    e. All of the above

20. According to recent evidence, which drug used to treat migraine headaches has some potential for addiction?
    a. tramadol (Ultram)
    b. chlorpromazine (Thorazine)
    c. ketorolac (Toradol)
    d. prochlorperazine (Compazine)

Chapter 7 Psychiatric and Related Drugs

Multiple Choice

Identify the choice that best completes the statement or answers the question.

1. Fluoxetine (Prozac) is an example of an antidepressant that appears to work through which of the following mechanisms?
   a. It inhibits the reuptake of serotonin into certain neurons in the brain.
   b. It blocks serotonin receptors in the limbic system.
   c. It is an agonist at alpha-2 adrenergic receptors throughout the central nervous system (CNS).
   d. It blocks muscarinic receptors and is a beta (nonselective) adrenergic receptor agonist.

2. Which antidepressant is a very versatile drug because it has three dosage forms?
   a. doxepin (Sinequan, Zonalon)
   b. maprotiline (Ludiomil)
   c. mirtazapine (Remeron)
   d. imipramine (Tofranil)

3. Which drug used to treat depression is also used for smoking cessation?
   a. trazodone (Desyrel)
   b. buproprion (Wellbutrin)
   c. carbamazepine (Tegretol)
   d. lithium (Lithobid)

4. What is the drug of choice for treating bipolar disorder and acute mania, and for prophylaxis of unipolar and bipolar disorders?
   a. valproic acid (Depakene)
   b. divalproex (Depakote)
   c. carbamazepine (Epitol, Tegretol)
   d. lithium (Eskalith, Lithobid)

5. What drug can be used as an alternative to lithium in the treatment of bipolar disorder, particularly with rapid cyclers?
   a. fluphenazine (Prolixin)
   b. escitalopram (Lexapro)
   c. maprotiline (Ludiomil)
   d. divalproex (Depakote)

6. Tardive dyskinesia is associated with the long-term use of which psychiatric medication?
   a. anticholinergics
   b. antipsychotics
   c. benzodiazepines
   d. SSRIs

7. Which of the following newer antipsychotic drugs is classified today as being "atypical"?
   a. molindone (Moban)
   b. haloperidol (Haldol)
   c. thiothixene (Navane)
   d. olanzapine (Zyprexa)

8. During which stages of sleep does dreaming occur?
   a. stages I and II
   b. stages I and IV
   c. stages III and IV
   d. By definition, dreaming occurs during all stages of sleep.

9. Which of the following drugs used to treat insomnia is *not* a DEA scheduled controlled substance?
   a. flurazepam (Dalmane)
   b. triazolam (Halcion)
   c. zolpidem (Ambien)
   d. diphenhydramine (Benadryl)

10. What class of drugs is part of the standard of care for alcohol (ethanol) detoxification?
    a. antipyretics
    b. antipsychotics
    c. benzodiazepines
    d. opiates

11. A characteristic of antidepressants is
    a. sedation lasting up to two weeks.
    b. delay in onset of relief from ten to twenty-one days.
    c. dependence if duration of therapy exceeds three months.
    d. adverse side effects for the first six weeks of therapy.

12. A child with a bed-wetting problem might be prescribed a(n)
    a. antianxiety agent.
    b. antipsychotic.
    c. tricyclic antidepressant.
    d. tetracyclic antidepressant.

13. Which class of antidepressants is second-line therapy because of interactions with foods and other drugs?
   a. SSRIs
   b. TCAs
   c. MAOIs
   d. SNRIs

14. Patients taking lithium must
   a. have blood tests regularly.
   b. take the medication two to three times daily at a specific time.
   c. avoid alcoholic beverages.
   d. keep their salt intake at a consistent level.
   e. All of the above

15. What is the primary indication for using antipsychotics?
   a. alcohol withdrawal
   b. panic disorder
   c. schizophrenia
   d. narcolepsy
   e. manic depression

16. Which mood-stabilizing drug has consistently been shown to decrease the risk of suicide for bipolar patients?
   a. haloperidol (Haldol)
   b. lithium (Eskalith, Lithobid)
   c. ziprasidone (Geodon)
   d. fluoxetine (Prozac)
   e. aripiprazole (Abilify)

17. Drugs that are used to treat psychotic disorders
   a. reverse memory impairment, confusion, and intellectual deterioration.
   b. improve emotional and social withdrawal.
   c. reduce thought disorders, hallucinations, and delusions.
   d. a and b
   e. a, b, and c

18. Why do most patients quit taking their antipsychotic medications?
   a. shortens the QT interval
   b. prolongs the QT interval
   c. weight gain
   d. hyperglycemia
   e. dyslipidemia

19. What percent of Americans who have trouble sleeping seek a physician's help?
   a. less than 10%
   b. 10 to 20%
   c. 21 to 30%
   d. 31 to 40%

20. Alcohol (ethanol) is classified as an
   a. anxiety agent.
   b. antidepressant.
   c. antiemetic.
   d. anesthetic.

Chapter 8 Drugs for Central Nervous System Disorders

Multiple Choice

Identify the choice that best completes the statement or answers the question.

1. What two neurotransmitters in the brain appear to play the greatest role in seizures?
   a. dopamine and GABA
   b. histamine and serotonin
   c. serotonin and glutamate
   d. GABA and glutamate

2. What term is used to describe continuous tonic-clonic seizures, lasting over 30 minutes, during which consciousness may not return?
   a. generalized seizures
   b. status epilepticus
   c. petit mal seizures
   d. grand mal seizures

3. What is the potential way in which antiepileptic medications can interact with each other and with other drugs?
   a. They can affect the absorption of other drugs.
   b. They can alter the metabolism of other drugs.
   c. They can alter the renal and hepatic distribution of other drugs.
   d. They can compete for transporters that affect drug access to the central nervous system (i.e., brain).
   e. all of the above

4. Which of the following anticonvulsants is a DEA scheduled controlled substance?
   a. carbamazepine (Tegretol)
   b. gabapentin (Neurontin)
   c. fosphenytoin (Cerebyx)
   d. phenytoin (Dilantin)
   e. diazepam (Valium)
5. The use of what anticonvulsant may result in physical or psychological dependence?
   a. levetriracetam (Keppra)
   b. ethosuximide (Zarontin)
   c. clonazepam (Klonopin)
   d. divalproex (Depakote)
6. Which anticonvulsant does *not* appear to act via GABA receptors and is frequently used to treat neuropathic pain?
   a. clonazepam (Klonopin)
   b. gabapentin (Neurontin)
   c. fosphenytoin (Cerebyx)
   d. topiramide (Topamax)
7. The prevalance of Parkinson disease (parkinsonism) is highest in what age group?
   a. newborns
   b. adolescents
   c. mid 30s to 40s
   d. mid 40s to 50
   e. above age 60
8. Which drug listed below is used to treat patients with multiple sclerosis?
   a. interferon beta-1a (Avonex, Rebif)
   b. interferon beta-1b (Betaseron)
   c. mitoxantrone (Novantrone)
   d. baclofen (Lioresal)
   e. All of the above
9. Which condition listed below is a chronic aching and stiffness with a lack of stamina?
   a. Huntington's Chorea
   b. Restless Leg Syndrome
   c. Fibromyalgia
   d. Parkinson's
10. Involuntary contractions or series of contractions of the voluntary muscles are called
    a. convolutions.
    b. conversions.
    c. convulsions.
    d. convictions.
    e. conveyances.
11. A generalized seizure
    a. is the most common type of seizure.
    b. occurs in two distinct types.
    c. involves both hemispheres of the brain simultaneously.
    d. may progress to a partial seizure.
12. Newer drugs for antiepileptic drug therapy
    a. have minimal adverse side effects.
    b. are recommended for polytherapy.
    c. have fewer drug interactions.
    d. are seizure-specific.
    e. have a wide therapeutic range.
13. What drug is both a prophylaxis and treatment for influenza, and is used to treat Parkinson disease?
    a. amantadine (Symmetrel)
    b. benztropine (Cogentin)
    c. ropinirole (ReQuip)
    d. pramipexole (Mirapex)
14. Which is a new class of anti-Parkinson agents that increase patient "on-time"?
    a. acetylcholinesterase inhibitors
    b. protease inhibitors
    c. catechol-o-methyl transferase inhibitors
    d. anistreplase inhibitors
15. What is a primary side effect of dextroamphetamine-amphetamine (Adderall)?
    a. bed-wetting in some children
    b. depression as the drug wears off
    c. weight gain and slow growth
    d. salivation
    e. nausea and vomiting
16. Which blood pressure medication is also used to treat ADD?
    a. atomoxetine (Strattera)
    b. baclofen (Lioresal)
    c. glatimer acetate (Copaxone)
    d. clonidine (Catapres)
17. Which of the following is part of the profile for Alzheimer disease?
    a. seizures
    b. depression
    c. severe trembling
    d. loss of overall muscle control
    e. blindness

18. Why might a prescribing physician prefer donepezil (Aricept) over tacrine (Cognex) for Alzheimer disease?
    a. Donepezil is given once a day.
    b. Donepezil does not result in nausea, vomiting, and diarrhea.
    c. Donepezil improves memory and alertness.
    d. a and b
    e. a, b, and c

19. What drug blocks NMDA (N-methyl-D-aspartate) in patients with Alzheimer disease?
    a. memantine (Namenda)
    b. donepezil (Aricept)
    c. galantamine (Razadyne)
    d. rivastigmine (Exelon)

20. What drug that is used to treat Alzheimer disease is derived from daffodil bulbs?
    a. rivastigmine (Exelon)
    b. tacrine (Cognex)
    c. galamtamine (Razadyne)
    d. memantine (Namenda)

Chapter 9 Respiratory Drugs

Multiple Choice

Identify the choice that best completes the statement or answers the question.

1. An asthma attack consists of how many phases or responses?
    a. 1
    b. 2
    c. 3
    d. 4

2. What is the most useful measure for assessing the severity of asthma?
    a. average inspiratory flow (AIF)
    b. median pulmonary retention rate (MPRR)
    c. peak expiratory flow rate (PEFR)
    d. pulmonary alveolar oxygen rate (PAOR)

3. What class of drugs used to treat hypertension, angina, cardiac arrhythmias, and migraine headaches is contraindicated in asthma patients?
    a. antihistamines
    b. beta blockers
    c. ACE inhibitors
    d. calcium channel blockers

4. Which of the following asthma medications blocks parasympathetic acetylcholine receptors and should *not* be given to patients with known peanut allergies?
    a. levalbuterol (Xopenex)
    b. aminophylline (Truphylline)
    c. zafirlukast (Accolate)
    d. ipratropium (Atrovent)
    e. fluticasone (Flonase, Flovent)

5. Which of the following medications is *least* likely to be used to treat or stop an acute asthma attack?
    a. albuterol (Proventil, Ventolin)
    b. epinephrine (EpiPen)
    c. terbutaline (Brethine)
    d. cromolyn sodium (Crolom, Gastrocrom)

6. Which of the following is an OTC expectorant available in caplet, capsule, liquid, syrup, tablet, and sustained-release forms?
    a. guaifenesin (Mucinex)
    b. pseudoephedrine (Sudafed)
    c. cetirizine (Zyrtec-D)
    d. ipratropium (Atrovent)
    e. loratadine (Claritin)

7. What is a potential symptom of nicotine withdrawal?
    a. anxiety
    b. difficulty in concentrating
    c. gastrointestinal disturbances
    d. increased appetite and weight gain
    e. All of the above

8. Why are many patients with asthma reluctant to use inhaled corticosteroids?
    a. They dislike the dosing regimen.
    b. They fear potential side effects.
    c. They object to the taste.
    d. They think corticosteroid inhalers are too difficult to use.

9. What is the chief criterion for diagnosing chronic bronchitis?
   a. how far the patient can walk without gasping for air
   b. how much sputum the patient produces over time
   c. whether or not the patient is overweight and has a barrel chest
   d. whether or not the patient has tachypnea

10. What is the best way for a patient with bronchitis to break up mucus and cough up secretions?
    a. take cough syrup
    b. use a mucolytic
    c. drink lots of water
    d. use a nebulizer
    e. tap on the lungs

11. What term is used for the major mechanism by which pulmonary pathogens gain access to the normally sterile lower airways and alveoli?
    a. aspiration
    b. expiration
    c. inspiration
    d. perspiration
    e. respiration

12. How long after exposure to tuberculosis is a patient most likely to show active symptoms of the disease?
    a. 4 to 10 weeks
    b. 1 to 2 years
    c. 5 years
    d. 20 years

13. In general, how many tuberculosis agents will be administered to a patient who has a positive TB skin test and a positive chest X-ray, but no symptoms?
    a. zero
    b. one
    c. two
    d. three
    e. four

14. Histoplasmosis is transmitted by
    a. having hand contact with an infected person.
    b. inhaling bacteria-laden drops.
    c. breathing in fungus-bearing dust.
    d. inheriting the gene for the disease from one's parents.

15. What are two types of receptors involved in the cough reflex?
    a. relaxed and spastic
    b. dilated and constricted
    c. smooth and striped
    d. stretch and irritant

16. Who should *not* take antihistamines?
    a. patients on a cruise
    b. patients having trouble sleeping
    c. patients taking antipsychotic medication
    d. pregnant patients
    e. patients with vertigo

17. Almost every OTC sleeping pill contains what antihistamine?
    a. diphenhydramine
    b. desloratadine
    c. hydroxyzine
    d. loratadine

18. What nasal corticosteroid may be used in children under 12 years of age?
    a. ciclesonide (Omnairs)
    b. mometasone (Nasonex)
    c. fluticasone (Flonase)
    d. a and c

19. Which dosage form most closely mimics the effects of cigarette smoking?
    a. nicotine nasal spray
    b. nicotine patch
    c. nicotine chewing gum
    d. nicotine lozenge

20. Which of the following gives correct instructions for using the nicotine patch?
    a. Apply a new patch weekly.
    b. Apply to a nonhairy, clean, dry site.
    c. Use the same application site.
    d. Apply to the lower body or outer leg.

Chapter 10 Drugs for Gastrointestinal and Related Diseases

Multiple Choice

Identify the choice that best completes the statement or answers the question.

1. Which drug listed below is an example of a phase II drug used to treat GERD?
   a. cimetidine (Tagamet)
   b. omeprazole (Prilosec)
   c. esomeprazole (Nexium)
   d. famotidine (Pepcid)
   e. All of the above

2. What group of drugs is the mainstay of treatment for *H. pylori*?
   a. antacids
   b. H_2 blockers
   c. antibiotics
   d. a and c
   e. All of the above

3. What is the drug of choice in treating malabsorption syndrome due to pancreatic insufficiency?
   a. sulfasalazine (Azulfidine)
   b. mesalamine (Asacol)
   c. infliximab (Remicade)
   d. pancrelipase (Creon-10)

4. Which of the drugs listed below is a monoclonal antibody that binds to tumor necrosis factor (TNF) and is indicated for the treatment of Crohn disease?
   a. olsalazine (Dipentum)
   b. infliximab (Remicade)
   c. metoclopramide (Reglan)
   d. esomeprazole (Nexium)

5. What effect does metoclopramide (Reglan) have as a prokinetic agent?
   a. It increases contraction in the G.I. tract
   b. It inhibits release of histamine in the GI tract.
   c. It is a prodrug, inactive until colon bacteria convert it.
   d. It dissolves cholesterol gallstones in the gallbladder.

6. Which drug or drug combination is *correctly* paired with its DEA control schedule?
   a. difenoxin-atropine (Motofen) - C-III
   b. diphenoxylate-atropine (Lomotil) - C-V
   c. nitazoxanide (Alinia) - C-IV
   d. rifaximin (Xifaxan) - not scheduled

7. Which medication below is used in preteens to treat diarrhea and acts by interfering with enzyme-dependent electron transfer in anaerobic energy metabolism?
   a. rifaximin (Xifaxan)
   b. polyethylene glycol (GoLYTELY)
   c. famotidine (Pepcid)
   d. nitazoxanide (Alinia)
   e. metoclopramide (Reglan)

8. What drug is metabolized by colonic bacteria and is used to prevent and treat hepatic-induced encephalopathy?
   a. bisacodyl (Dulcolax)
   b. magnesium hydroxide (Milk of Magnesia)
   c. bismuth subsalicylate (Pepto-Bismol)
   d. lactulose (Enulose)

9. Which drug listed below acts to facilitate the admixture of fat and water to soften stool?
   a. psyllium (Metamucil)
   b. bisacodyl (Dulcolax)
   c. simethicone (Mylanta)
   d. docusate-senna (Senokot-S)

10. Which of the following drugs is used for chemotherapy-induced emesis and frequently causes headaches in patients treated with it?
    a. ondansetron (Zofran)
    b. sibutramine (Meridia)
    c. primaquine
    d. prochlorperazine (Compazine)

11. What is praziquantel (Biltricide) used to treat?
    a. intestinal parasites (tapeworms)
    b. amebiasis caused by *Entamoeba histolytica*
    c. malaria
    d. hepatitis

12. What drug has been used since the seventeenth century and is now used in combination with other drugs to treat malaria?
    a. quinine (Qualaquin)
    b. mefloquine (Lariam)
    c. doxycycline (Vibramycin)
    d. chloroquine (Aralen)

13. Who is likely to be bothered by GERD?
    a. a pregnant patient
    b. a patient with a hiatal hernia
    c. an overweight patient
    d. a patient with poor eating habits
    e. All of the above

14. Which of the following is used as phase I medication to treat GERD?
    a. proton pump inhibitors
    b. antacids
    c. coating agents
    d. cholinergic agents
    e. H_2 receptor antagonists

15. Antimotility medications are used to treat
    a. chronic diarrhea.
    b. short-term constipation.
    c. acute malabsorption.
    d. terminal gastritis.

16. What drug is used to treat traveler's diarrhea?
    a. nitazoxanide (Alinia)
    b. diphenoxylate-atropine (Lomotil)
    c. ursodiol (Actigall)
    d. rifaximin (Xifaxan)

17. Which drug is a lipase inhibitor used to treat obesity?
    a. orlistat (Xenical)
    b. sibutramine (Meridia)
    c. diethylpropion (Tenuate)
    d. phentermine (Ionamin)

18. Which of the following is used to treat tapeworm infestation and microsporidiasis?
    a. thiabendazole (Mintezol)
    b. albendazole (Albenza)
    c. mebendazole (Vermox)
    d. praziquantel (Biltricide)

19. What are protozoa?
    a. animals that live in the bodies of other animals
    b. organisms that function as intermediate hosts
    c. single-cell organisms that inhabit soil and water
    d. worms that live in human and animal intestines

20. A protozoan found in the human intestine and the cause of many GI infections is
    a. trichinella.
    b. giardia.
    c. ascaris.
    d. strongyloide.

Chapter 11 Renal System Drugs

Multiple Choice

Identify the choice that best completes the statement or answers the question.

1. What term is used to describe the working units of the kidneys?
    a. glomeruli
    b. renin
    c. nephrons
    d. filtrons

2. What do the kidneys regulate?
    a. blood plasma volume
    b. concentration of waste products in the blood
    c. electrolyte concentrations
    d. plasma acid-base balance
    e. All of the above

3. What is *not* one of the processes by which the kidneys produce urine?
    a. filtration
    b. reabsorption
    c. secretion
    d. induction

4. What is a goal of renal therapy?
   a. reestablishing an appropriate intravascular volume
   b. restricting fluids in volume-overload patients
   c. treating underlying fluid, electrolyte, or pH problems
   d. All of the above
5. What hormone is diminished in patients with anemia due to renal failure?
   a. hematocrit
   b. erythropoietin
   c. pyridoxine
   d. renin
6. What is the first oral therapy for interstitial cystitis?
   a. bethanechol (Urecholine)
   b. methenamine (Cystex, Hiprex, Urex)
   c. pentosan polysulfate sodium (Elmiron)
   d. mycophenolic acid (Myfortic)
7. Which of the following agents for urinary tract problems is available OTC?
   a. flavoxate (Urispas)
   b. oxybutynin (Ditropan)
   c. tolterodine (Detrol)
   d. phenazopyridine (Azo-Standard, Uristat)
8. What antibiotic (or combination) may be used to treat urinary tract infections (UTIs)?
   a. amoxicillin (Amoxil, Trimox)
   b. amoxicillin-clavulanate (Augmentin)
   c. ciprofloxacin (Cipro)
   d. nitrofurantoin (Macrobid, Macrodantin)
   e. All of the above
9. What class of drugs is commonly used to treat benign prostatic hyperplasia (BPH)?
   a. alpha blockers
   b. tricyclic antidepressants
   c. antihistamines
   d. penicillins
10. Who should never handle crushed tablets of finasteride (Propecia, Proscar)?
   a. adolescents
   b. pregnant women
   c. men with BPH
   d. children
11. What is the function of the ureter?
   a. to regulate the concentration of waste products in urine
   b. to conduct urine from the kidneys to the bladder
   c. to exchange potassium in the urine for sodium
   d. to collect urine until it is released from the body
   e. to conduct urine from the bladder to outside of the body
12. In which part of the urine-producing process are filtered substances selectively pulled back into the blood?
   a. filtration
   b. reabsorption
   c. secretion
   d. induction
13. What might be a sign of stage 2 renal disease?
   a. anorexia
   b. nocturia
   c. pruritus
   d. metabolic acidosis
   e. hypocalcemia
14. What is a sign that inhibiting substances are being removed by dialysis?
   a. decline in hematocrit
   b. rise in hematocrit
   c. decline in hematite
   d. rise in hemolymph
15. What is an advantage of mycophenolate (CellCept), an immunosuppressant?
   a. It comes in only a tablet form.
   b. It comes in only an oral liquid form.
   c. It comes in an injection form.
   d. It comes in an IV form.
16. Which group has the highest incidence of urinary tract infections?
   a. older men
   b. sexually active women
   c. bed-wetting children
   d. athletes
   e. postmenopausal women

17. Which of the following is a urinary tract infection of the upper tract?
    a. cystitis
    b. urethritis
    c. prostatitis
    d. pyelonephritis
18. Which of these do prescribers sometimes recommend for patients taking methenamine (Cystex, Hiprex, Urex)?
    a. cranberry juice
    b. orange juice
    c. antacids
    d. bicarbonate
19. Benign prostatic hyperplasia (BPH) becomes a problem when
    a. cancerous cells are unresponsive to treatment.
    b. secretion of prostatic antibacterial factor is slowed.
    c. urine flow from the bladder is obstructed.
    d. urine from the ureter to the bladder is obstructed.
20. Which class of diuretics should be prescribed with caution to patients on ACE inhibitors?
    a. thiazides
    b. loops
    c. potassium-sparing
    d. carbonic anhydrase inhibitors
    e. osmotics

Chapter 12 Drugs for Cardiovascular Diseases

Multiple Choice

Identify the choice that best completes the statement or answers the question.

1. What term describes the electrical signal that causes a muscle to contract?
    a. depolarization
    b. action potential
    c. repolarization
    d. ion flow
2. What are two lifestyle factors that may contribute to the development of heart disease?
    a. hereditary and cigarette smoking
    b. gender and increasing age
    c. high blood pressure and gender
    d. obesity and cigarette smoking
3. Which of the following drug classes is *not* used to treat angina?
    a. nitrates
    b. beta blockers
    c. calcium channel blockers
    d. angiotensin II receptor antagonists
4. Which of the following is a beta blocker that is commonly used in the treatment of angina?
    a. ranolozine (Ranexa)
    b. verapamil (Calan)
    c. nicardipine (Cardene)
    d. acebutolol (Sectral)
5. What antiarrhythmic agent is also an anticonvulsant agent?
    a. dofetilide (Tikosyn)
    b. procainamide (Procanbid, Pronestyl)
    c. digoxin (Lanoxicaps, Lanoxin)
    d. phenytoin (Dilantin)
6. What term describes a thickening of the heart muscle in an enlarged heart?
    a. cardioversion
    b. cardiomegaly
    c. myocardial hypertrophy
    d. myocardial infarction (MI)
7. Which of the following is a central nervous system agent used to treat hypertension?
    a. guanfacine (Tenex)
    b. losartan (Cozaar)
    c. minoxidil (Loniten)
    d. doxazosin (Cardura)
8. Which of the following antihypertensive drugs is an antiotension II receptor antagonist?
    a. valsartan (Diovan)
    b. benazepril (Lotensin)
    c. prazosin (Minipress)
    d. propranolol (Inderal)

9. Beta blockers may be used in combination with what other drug to reduce the risk of death or recurrence following a myocardial infarction?
   a. digoxin (Lanoxin)
   b. atenolol (Tenormin)
   c. aspirin
   d. bismuth subsalicylate
10. Which of the following anticoagulant drugs is available in tablet form?
   a. heparin
   b. bivalirudin (Angiomax)
   c. dalteparin (Fragmin)
   d. warfarin (Coumadin)
11. Which of the following drugs used for MIs and stroke prevention blocks ADP receptors, reducing platelet adhesion and aggregation?
   a. aspirin
   b. clopidogrel (Plavix)
   c. pentoxifylline (Trental)
   d. dipyridamole (Persantine)
12. Which of the antiplatelet drugs listed below is a monoclonal antibody?
   a. abciximab (ReoPro)
   b. eptifibatide (Integrilin)
   c. tirofiban (Aggrastat)
   d. clopidogrel (Plavix)
13. If circulation of oxygen to the brain is stopped, how long will it take for the brain to use up its supply of oxygen?
   a. 5 seconds
   b. 10 seconds
   c. 15 seconds
   d. 20 seconds
14. Why do most statins work better if taken in the evening?
   a. Patients are more likely to remember to take them.
   b. They can cause GI disturbances.
   c. Most cholesterol is produced at night.
   d. Most cholesterol is produced during the day.
15. What term refers to an abnormally slow heart rate?
   a. arrhythmia
   b. bradycardia
   c. hypoglycemia
   d. hypertension
16. Congestive heart failure is characterized by the accumulation of fluid in the body tissues, or
   a. eczema.
   b. edema.
   c. eclampsia.
   d. enema.
17. Diuretics help to lower blood pressure by
   a. reducing preload.
   b. increasing preload.
   c. reducing afterload.
   d. increasing afterload.
18. Which laboratory test indicates the proportion of the blood sample that is red blood cells?
   a. partial thromboplastin time
   b. prothrombin time
   c. International Normalized Ratio
   d. hematocrit
19. Which organ of the body is responsible for making new cholesterol when needed?
   a. pancreas
   b. kidneys
   c. large intestine
   d. liver
   e. gall bladder
20. Patients with hyperlipidemia should avoid
   a. estrogen.
   b. calcium channel blockers.
   c. loop diuretics.
   d. clonidine.

Chapter 13 Drugs for Muscle and Joint Disease and Pain

Multiple Choice

Identify the choice that best completes the statement or answers the question.

1. What muscle relaxant is a scheduled substance in many states due to its potential for abuse?
   a. metaxalone (Skelaxin)
   b. orphenadrine (Norflex)
   c. chlorzoxazone (Paraflex)
   d. carisoprodol (Soma)

2. Which of the following muscle relaxants acts on benzodiazepine receptors?
   a. dantrolene (Dantrium)
   b. diazepam (Valium)
   c. methocarbamol (Robaxin)
   d. orphenadrine (Norflex)

3. What substances reduce pain, fever, and inflammation?
   a. synovia
   b. salicylates
   c. tophi
   d. analgesics

4. How do salicylates reduce fever?
   a. increasing blood flow to skin and inhibiting PG synthesis
   b. decreasing blood flow to skin and inhibiting PG synthesis
   c. increasing blood flow to hypothalamus
   d. decreasing blood flow to hypothalamus

5. Why should aspirin *not* be given to children?
   a. It may cause salicylism in children.
   b. It increases the risk of developing chicken pox in children.
   c. Reye syndrome can develop in children who have been exposed to chicken pox.
   d. It can cause irreversible bleeding problems in children.

6. What prostaglandin molecule, which facilitates platelet aggregation, is inhibited by low dose (81-325 mg) aspirin?
   a. thromboxane A_2
   b. prostacyclin
   c. PGE2
   d. cyclooxygenase

7. What clinical effect or side effect of aspirin is also produced by acetaminophen (Tylenol)?
   a. fever reduction
   b. GI irritation
   c. altered platelet adhesion and bleeding
   d. inflammation reduction

8. NSAIDs can interact with which of the following drug classes?
   a. antibiotics
   b. beta adrenergic agonists
   c. oral hypoglycemics
   d. antacids

9. Which of the following drugs is *least* likely to produce GI irritation at analgesic doses?
   a. naproxen (Aleve, Anaprox, Naprosyn)
   b. sulindac (Clinoril)
   c. aspirin
   d. celecoxib (Celebrex)

10. What ties one bone to another bone?
    a. myofibril
    b. muscles
    c. ligaments
    d. tendons

11. Which of the following begins the process of muscle contraction?
    a. calcium
    b. ACh
    c. sodium ions
    d. potassium

12. What warning label should appear on prescriptions for muscle relaxants?
    a. May cause drowsiness.
    b. This drug interferes with the effectiveness of oral contraceptives.
    c. Do not take if pregnant.
    d. Refrigerate after opening.
    e. May turn urine blue.

13. An unlabeled use for baclofen (Lioresal) is for treating
    a. multiple sclerosis.
    b. reversible spasticity.
    c. spinal cord lesions.
    d. hiccups.

14. Why might dantrolene (Dantrium) be used in the operating room?
    a. to reverse a narcotic overdose
    b. to sedate patients prior to surgery
    c. to treat malignant hyperthermia
    d. to facilitate endotracheal intubation

15. What nonnarcotic analgesic can be prescribed in the dosage form of gum?
    a. acetaminophen (Tylenol)
    b. acetylcysteine (Mucomyst)
    c. salsalate (Amigesic)
    d. aspirin

16. Which type of arthritis results in loss of cartilage elasticity and thickness and causes bone to wear and become deformed?
    a. osteoarthritis
    b. bursitis
    c. rheumatoid arthritis
    d. gouty arthritis
17. Rheumatoid arthritis is usually symmetric, which means that the
    a. fingers become immobile and clawlike.
    b. same joints on both sides of the body are affected.
    c. small joints of the hand are affected first.
    d. vertebral column becomes stiff and painful.
18. In the near future, more NSAIDs are expected
    a. to be available by prescription only.
    b. to become controlled substances.
    c. to be sold over the counter.
    d. to be classified as DMARDs.
19. Which NSAID has an oral liquid form and is suitable for children?
    a. naproxen (Aleve)
    b. ibuprofen (Advil, Motrin)
    c. mefenamic acid (Ponstel)
    d. etodolac (Lodine)
    e. buffered aspirin (Bufferin)
20. What causes gouty arthritis?
    a. improper excretion of uric acid
    b. long-term elevated LDL cholesterol levels
    c. chronic hypertension
    d. abnormal activity by chondrocytes, or cartilage cells

Chapter 14 Hormonal Disorders and Their Treatment

Multiple Choice

Identify the choice that best completes the statement or answers the question.

1. What is the drug of choice for chronic thyroid treatment?
    a. levothyroxine (Levothroid, Synthroid)
    b. thyroid (Armour Thyroid)
    c. methimazole (Tapazole)
    d. a and b
2. Which of the following drugs or drug classes may cause male impotence?
    a. alcohol
    b. corticosteroids
    c. haloperidol (Haldol)
    d. opiates
    e. All of the above
3. Which of the following drugs is used for emergency contraception?
    a. ethinyl estradiol-drospirenone (Yasmin)
    b. levonorgestrel (Plan B)
    c. estradiol cypionate-medroxyprogesterone (Lunelle)
    d. estradiol (Estrace, Vivelle)
    e. ethinyl drospirenone (Angeliq)
4. Which of the following drugs may interact adversely with oral contraceptives?
    a. erythromycin
    b. carbamazepine
    c. prednisolone
    d. clofibrate
    e. All of the above
5. Which of the following drugs is used to treat genital herpes?
    a. acyclovir (Zovirax)
    b. doxycycline (Vibramycin)
    c. penicillin G benzathine (Bicillin L-A)
    d. clotrimazole (GyneLotrimin, Mycelex)
    e. tertacycline (Sumycin)

6. What is *not* a potential adverse effect of corticosteroids?
   a. hypotension due to increased sodium excretion
   b. cataracts
   c. increased susceptibility to infections
   d. osteoporosis

7. Which synthetic insulin is the longest acting?
   a. lispro (Humalog)
   b. aspart (Novolog)
   c. NPH (Humulin N)
   d. glargine (Lantus)

8. Which structure releases hormones that regulate secondary sex characteristics?
   a. testes
   b. adrenal glands
   c. pituitary gland
   d. eyes
   e. a, b, and c

9. What is hypogonadism?
   a. deficient sex hormone production and secretion
   b. development of male characteristics
   c. development of female characteristics
   d. painful penile erections

10. What is the advantage of a scrotal transdermal system in treating hypogonadism?
    a. It mimics the natural circadian secretion of serum testosterone.
    b. It avoids first-pass metabolism in the gastrointestinal tract.
    c. It is painless and easy to apply.
    d. a and b
    e. a, b, and c

11. Hormone replacement therapy is controversial because it is associated with increased risk of
    a. osteoporosis.
    b. cardiovascular disease.
    c. breast cancer.
    d. memory loss.
    e. All of the above

12. Combined estrogen-progestin oral contraceptives prevent conception by
    a. interfering with the production of the hormones that regulate the menstrual cycle.
    b. altering the cervical mucus to form a physical barrier that prevents the penetration of sperm.
    c. changing the composition of the endometrium to make it unsuitable for implantation.
    d. a and b
    e. a, b, and c

13. Which of the following can yield a false-positive result with a home pregnancy test?
    a. collecting the urine in a waxed paper cup
    b. using a refrigerated sample that has been warmed
    c. diluting the urine
    d. b and c
    e. All of the above

14. Which agent is used for uncontrolled bleeding at childbirth?
    a. oxytocin (Pitocin)
    b. norgestrel (Ovrette)
    c. medroxyprogesterone (Depo-Provera)
    d. methylergonovine (Methergine)

15. What is needed for calcium to absorb into bone tissue?
    a. vitamin A
    b. vitamin B
    c. vitamin C
    d. vitamin D
    e. vitamin E

16. Which structure of the endocrine system releases cortisol into the blood?
    a. pituitary gland
    b. hypothalamus
    c. adrenal glands
    d. thyroid gland
    e. ovaries

17. The specialized cells responsible for producing insulin are located in the
    a. liver.
    b. kidneys.
    c. pancreas.
    d. gall bladder.
    e. stomach.

18. Acute hypoglycemia occurs when
    a. plasma glucose is above 600 mg/dL of blood.
    b. blood glucose levels two hours after eating are 200–400 mg/dL.
    c. fasting glucose is 80–120 mg/dL of blood.
    d. blood glucose levels fall below 70 mg/dL.
19. A patient with diabetes might take a statin to
    a. control blood pressure.
    b. manage cholesterol levels.
    c. help cells use glucose more efficiently.
    d. prevent gluconeogenesis.
20. Who is most likely to benefit from growth hormone (GH) replacement?
    a. male, age 10
    b. female, age 14
    c. male in whom epiphyseal closure has occurred
    d. child with Down syndrome

Chapter 15 Topical, Ophthalmic, and Otic Medications

Multiple Choice

Identify the choice that best completes the statement or answers the question.

1. What is the top layer of skin known as?
    a. ectoderm
    b. endoderm
    c. epidermis
    d. None of the above
2. What term is used to describe the excessive response of the skin to sun in the presence of a sensitizing agent?
    a. photoreactivity
    b. photosensitivity
    c. photoconductivity
    d. acne
3. Which of the following drugs is *not* used to treat fungal infections?
    a. butenafine (Lotrimin Ultra, Mentax)
    b. clotrimazole (Lotrimin)
    c. tolnaftate (Tinactin)
    d. fluorouracil (Efudex)
4. What is the most common allergic reaction to a drug?
    a. hives
    b. diarrhea
    c. nausea
    d. rash
5. What features are characteristic of rosacea?
    a. redness, warmth, local pain, and plaque
    b. flushing, erythema, papules, and pustules
    c. red, scaly skin and arthritis
    d. erythema, edema, and vesicles
6. Which of the following drugs, derived from chrysanthemums, is available OTC and is used for head lice?
    a. lindane
    b. pyrethrins (Rid Mousse)
    c. permethrin (Elimite, Nix)
    d. betamethasone dipropionate (Diprosone)
7. What drug applied topically for wound healing works by stimulating the growth of collagen fibroblasts?
    a. phenytoin (Dilantin)
    b. crotamiton (Eurax)
    c. chlorhexidine gluconate (Hibiclens)
    d. carbamide peroxide (Gly-Oxide Oral)
8. What drug is used to treat cytomegalovirus (CMV), an inflammation of the retina that is caused by a virus?
    a. ketotifen (Zaditor)
    b. ganciclovir (Vitrasert)
    c. verteporfin (Visudyne)
    d. cyclosporine (Restasis)
9. What causes age-related macular degeneration (AMD)?
    a. excessive sun exposure
    b. adverse reaction to antibiotics
    c. infection
    d. unknown
10. What drug is used to treat chronic keratoconjunctivitis (dry eye)?
    a. cyclosporine (Restasis)
    b. loteprednol (Alrex, Lotemax)
    c. ketotifen (Zaditor)
    d. olopatadine (Patanol)

11. Which of the following is an eardrop?
    a. apraclonidine (Iopidine)
    b. betaxolol (Betoptic)
    c. echothiophate iodide (Phospholine Iodide)
    d. antipyrine-benzocaine (Auralgan)

12. Which drug used to treat glaucoma may cause light-colored eyes to turn brown?
    a. latanoprost (Xalatan)
    b. dorzolamide (Trusopt)
    c. apraclonidine (Iopidine)
    d. brinzolamide (Azopt)

13. Sunburn greatly increases the risk of what skin disorder?
    a. squamous cell carcinoma
    b. melanoma
    c. basal cell carcinoma
    d. keratoacanthoma

14. Local freezing can be used to treat
    a. dandruff.
    b. warts.
    c. unwanted facial hair.
    d. ringworm.
    e. actinic keratosis.

15. Eflornithine (Vaniqa)
    a. is approved to be used only by men.
    b. is approved to be used only by women.
    c. has no known side effects.
    d. should be applied three times daily.

16. Which of the following skin disorders is a fungal infection?
    a. dandruff
    b. cellulitis
    c. psoriasis
    d. candidiasis
    e. dermatitis

17. Which class of drugs is typically used to treat poison ivy?
    a. antibiotics
    b. corticosteroids
    c. antihistamines
    d. antivirals

18. Open-angle glaucoma is usually treated with
    a. eyedrops.
    b. laser surgery.
    c. intravitreal injection.
    d. oral agents.

19. Which oral agent is used to treat glaucoma and is also used for altitude sickness?
    a. lantanoprost (Xalatan)
    b. brinzolamide (Azopt)
    c. bimatoprost (Lumigan)
    d. aclometasone (Aclovate)

20. The pharmacy technician should inform the pharmacist if
    a. the physician prescribes eardrops for an eye infection.
    b. the physician prescribes an otic antibiotic but not an accompanying pain reliever.
    c. the physician prescribes an otic solution for a patient with a tube in the ear.
    d. a and b
    e. a, b, and c

Chapter 16 Recombinant Drugs and Chemotherapy

Multiple Choice

Identify the choice that best completes the statement or answers the question.

1. Which of the following drugs may be given to suppress infection and increase the production of white blood cells in patients receiving chemotherapy?
    a. pegfilgrastim (Neulasta)
    b. interferon beta-1a (Avonex, Rebif)
    c. interferon beta-1b (Betaseron)
    d. dornase alfa (Pulmozyme)

2. Which of the following drugs is produced using recombinant DNA technology?
    a. flutamide (Eulexin)
    b. cyclosporine (Sandimmune)
    c. aldesleukin (Proleukin)
    d. tamoxifen (Nolvadex)
    e. All of the above

3. Which of the following interferons is used to treat multiple sclerosis?
    a. interferon beta-1b (Betaseron)
    b. interferon alfa-2a (Roferon A)
    c. interferon alfa-2b (Intron A)
    d. All of the above

4. T cells and B cells both arise from the
   a. liver.
   b. thymus.
   c. bone marrow.
   d. spleen.
5. Which immunity process is responsible for organ transplant rejection and hypersensitivity reactions?
   a. humoral
   b. cellular
   c. lymphatic
   d. opsonization
6. What is the purpose of the lymphatic system?
   a. to maintain the balance of water, electrolytes, and acids and bases in the extra-cellular fluid
   b. to detect the presence of chemicals in the body and convert that information into a chemical/electrical message
   c. to filter body fluids by nodes, vessels, and lymphocytes before the fluids return to general circulation
   d. to produce secretions that are responsible for specific regulatory effects on organs and other tissues of the body
7. Which immunoglobulin is the most commonly used in the production of MAbs?
   a. IgA
   b. IgD
   c. IgE
   d. IgG
   e. IgM
8. How would a pharmacy technician know that a drug is a monoclonal antibody?
   a. The name of the drug ends in "ine".
   b. The name of the drug ends in "mab".
   c. The name of the drug ends in "cin".
   d. The name of the drug ends in "mus".
9. What drug is used to treat Hodgkin disease?
   a. imatinib (Gleevec)
   b. gefitnib (Iressa)
   c. pemetrexad (Alimta)
   d. procarbazine (Matulane)
10. What drug combination is known as "Magic Swizzle"?
    a. phenol-sodium borate-sodium bicarbonate-glycerin
    b. chlorhexidine gluconate
    c. lidocaine-diphenhydramine-Maalox
    d. phenol-sodium borate-sodium bicarbonate-glycerin
11. The final step in the natural process for making proteins is
    a. copying.
    b. transcription.
    c. replication.
    d. translation.
12. What is the part of DNA where protein production starts?
    a. promoter sequence
    b. terminator sequence
    c. RNA polymerase
    d. nucleotide bases
13. Which class of recombinant DNA drugs is used to influence the bone marrow to produce blood cells?
    a. colony-stimulating factor
    b. biologic-response modifier
    c. fibrinolytic agent
    d. secretion-thinning enzyme
    e. hematologic agent
14. Which drug is a rescue agent?
    a. interferon beta-1a (Avonex, Rebif)
    b. antihemophilic factor (Alphanate)
    c. leucovorin
    d. sargramostim (Leukine)
15. Which immunoglobulin is the main Ig in salivary and bronchial secretions?
    a. IgG
    b. IgM
    c. IgA
    d. IgE
    e. IgD
16. Monoclonal antibodies medications are administered in what dosage forms?
    a. IV, capsule
    b. IV, tablet
    c. IV, injection
    d. IV, injection, oral liquid
17. Which antirejection drug is a monoclonal antibody?

a. cyclosporine (Sandimmune)
b. basiliximab (Simulect)
c. mycophenolate (CellCept)
d. tacrolimus (Prograf)

18. Which of the following is true of cancer cells?
 a. Cancer cells have no useful function.
 b. Cancer cells develop and reproduce at a faster rate than normal cells.
 c. Cancer cells possess contact inhibition.
 d. a and b
 e. a, b, and c

19. Antitumor drugs are
 a. most efficient when tumor cells are dividing rapidly.
 b. extremely toxic.
 c. periodically stopped for two to six weeks.
 d. a and c
 e. a, b, and c

20. Which of the following cytoprotective drugs is used to reduce the side effects and toxicity of chemotherapy agents?
 a. amifostine (Ethyol)
 b. dexrazoxane (Zinecard)
 c. leucovorin
 d. All of the above

Chapter 17 Vitamins, OTC Supplements, Antidotes, and Miscellaneous Topics

Multiple Choice

Identify the choice that best completes the statement or answers the question.

1. What organ maintains the largest stores of fat-soluble vitamins?
 a. small intestines
 b. liver
 c. kidneys
 d. spleen

2. What are the symptoms of vitamin B_3, or niacin, deficiency?
 a. diarrhea, dementia, dermatitis
 b. muscle weakness, diarrhea
 c. inability to walk, muscle weakness
 d. dementia, cataracts, weakened immune system

3. What can restore or promote the growth of normal bacterial flora in the body?
 a. vitamin B_7
 b. vitamin E
 c. flavocoxid (Limbrel)
 d. probiotics
 e. potassium

4. What form of calcium is most commonly used in cardiac emergencies?
 a. calcium chloride
 b. calcium carbonate
 c. calcium acetate
 d. calcium gluconate

5. In what type of solution are there fewer particles (that is, a lower concentration) than contained in body fluids?
 a. hypotonic
 b. isotonic
 c. hypertonic
 d. catatonic

6. What term describes a method in which the patient is fed through a vein?
 a. enteral nutrition
 b. total parenteral nutrition
 c. peroral nutrition
 d. None of the above

7. Which of the following drugs may cause tinnitus (ringing in the ear), nausea, and vomiting in children with doses greater than 150 mg/kg?
 a. tricyclic antidepressants
 b. aspirin
 c. morphine
 d. acetaminophen (Tylenol)

8. What drug may be used to treat drug-induced bradycardia?
 a. digoxin immune Fab (Digibind)
 b. atropine
 c. naloxone (Narcan)
 d. penicillamine (Cuprimine)

9. What reversal agent may be used to treat narcotic respiratory depression?
   a. edetate calcium disodium (Calcium Disodium Versenate)
   b. phentolamine (Regitine)
   c. naloxone (Narcan)
   d. glucagon (GlucaGen)

10. What toxin with the potential for bioterrorism is derived from the castor bean?
   a. atropine
   b. botulin
   c. tuberemia
   d. anthrax
   e. ricin

11. A deficiency of vitamin C may lead to
   a. keratomalacia.
   b. rickets.
   c. beriberi.
   d. pellagra.
   e. scurvy.

12. What is another name for vitamin B_9?
   a. thiamine
   b. riboflavin
   c. nicotinic acid
   d. pyridoxine
   e. folic acid

13. Proportionally, who has the highest amount of body water?
   a. a lean, well-muscled male adult
   b. an obese adult
   c. an adult female
   d. an elderly person
   e. a newborn

14. What is a sign of malnutrition?
   a. poor wound healing
   b. increased number of infections
   c. breathing difficulties
   d. anemia
   e. All of the above

15. Which is correct for preparing a TPN solution?
   a. Add the vitamins when the mixture is initially prepared.
   b. Add the vitamins just before administration.
   c. Add the vitamins and then put in the electrolytes.
   d. Add the vitamins before the amino acids, dextrose, lipids, and water.

16. In contrast to two-in-ones, three-in-one TPN solutions
   a. are more stable and thus last longer.
   b. allow precipitants to be easily seen.
   c. may crack or separate.
   d. can remain at room temperature for forty-eight hours.

17. Which of the following is the leading cause of fatal poisonings in children?
   a. mouthwash
   b. antidepressants
   c. iron tablets
   d. aspirin

18. What is the most common route for poisoning?
   a. injection
   b. skin contamination
   c. inhalation
   d. ingestion

19. What is the treatment for a black widow spider bite in a healthy adult?
   a. an antivenin
   b. supportive therapy
   c. dapsone
   d. a and b
   e. a, b, and c

20. What may be a pharmacy technician's duty in the event of a bioterrorism attack?
   a. joining the response team
   b. identifying patient allergies
   c. dispensing drugs
   d. keeping records
   e. All of the above

Unit Tests

Unit 1 Introduction to Pharmacology

Multiple Choice

Identify the choice that best completes the statement or answers the question.

1. What organization was established in 1852 to counter the encroachment of other medical areas into pharmacy?
   a. American Medical Association (AMA)
   b. American Pharmaceutical Association (APhA)
   c. Pharmaceutical Manufacturers of America (PMA)
   d. International Association of Formulators and Dispensers (IAFD)

2. What is another term for a drug's United States Adopted Name (USAN)?
   a. chemical
   b. generic
   c. trade
   d. brand

3. What action did the FDA take to speed up the approval of urgently needed drugs?
   a. It instituted the Prescription Drug User Fee Act.
   b. It reduced the number of patients required to participate in phase III of clinical trials.
   c. It allowed pharmaceutical manufacturers (sponsors) to test a new drug's safety and efficacy without FDA oversight.
   d. It partially reduced the scope of phase IV clinical studies.

4. Drugs from which FDA Pregnancy Category can safely be used in pregnant patients?
   a. A
   b. B
   c. C
   d. D
   e. X

5. What is *not* true of FDA-approved generic drugs?
   a. They must contain the same active ingredients as the original drug.
   b. Although they may have a new generic name or USAN, generic drugs may keep the trade name of the original drug.
   c. Generic drugs must be identical in strength, dosage form, and route of administration to the original drug.
   d. They must have the same indications as the original drug.

6. Manufacturers of foods containing which ingredients may make health claims regarding the disease-fighting action of the food?
   a. whole grains
   b. simple carbohydrates
   c. unsaturated fats
   d. gluten
   e. low fat

7. Which of the following was a major pharmacological advance during the Middle Ages?
   a. administering drugs topically, orally, and rectally
   b. making drugs from chemical substances
   c. associating plants with the disease they were intended to treat
   d. using individual drugs rather than mixtures or potions

8. What event forced American physicians and druggists to make their own drugs?
   a. French and Indian War
   b. American Revolution
   c. War of 1812
   d. Civil War
   e. World War I

9. Who developed the first effective treatment for diabetes?
   a. Sir Alexander Fleming
   b. Gerhardt Domagk
   c. Sir Frederick Banting and Charles Best
   d. Ignaz Philip Semmelweis
   e. Paul Ehrlich

10. Which task might a pharmacy technician in a hospital pharmacy perform?
    a. prepare sterile IVs and chemotherapy compounds
    b. conduct a "tech check tech" in the preparation of medicine carts
    c. educate nurses about pharmacy-related issues
    d. a and c
    e. a, b, and c

11. When was the law passed that established two classes of drugs?
    a. 1927
    b. 1938
    c. 1951
    d. 1953

12. Professionals and consumers can report serious adverse drug reactions to
    a. MedWatch.
    b. the DEA.
    c. the USP-NF.
    d. the PTCB.
    e. the NABP.

13. A Black Box warning
    a. alerts prescribers to the known problems with the use of the drug.
    b. allows the prescriber to weigh the advantage of using this drug with its risks.
    c. is on thousands of drugs on the market.
    d. a, b, and c

14. A rating system devised by the FDA to establish the therapeutic equivalent of generic drugs is the
    a. pass/fail system.
    b. +/− system.
    c. thumbs-up system.
    d. one/two system.
    e. A/B system.

15. What should pharmacy technicians do when helping patients select OTC products?
    a. point out price differentials
    b. check the control schedule
    c. read the ingredients
    d. recommend brand names

16. What term is used to describe the strength by which a particular messenger binds to its receptor site?
    a. agonist
    b. antagonist
    c. potency
    d. affinity

17. What is the study of the activity of drugs within the body known as?
    a. pharmacodynamics
    b. pharmacokinetics
    c. pharmacology
    d. pharmacognosy

18. In what way are the capillaries in the central nervous system (CNS) different from other capillaries?
    a. They contain double membranes, making it more difficult for lipid-soluble drugs to enter the CNS.
    b. They lack essential drug transporters necessary to distribute drugs into the CNS.
    c. They are enveloped by glial cells, which are additional barriers against water-soluble compounds.
    d. Except for sedatives and analgesics, the meninges must be disturbed before other drugs can enter the CNS.

19. What is a classic example of a drug that is eliminated by a zero-order pharmacokinetic process?
    a. alcohol
    b. aspirin
    c. penicillin
    d. nicotine
    e. All of the above

20. What is a common side effect of narcotics?
    a. swelling
    b. constipation
    c. wheals
    d. wheezing

21. How does grapefruit juice interact with certain drugs?
  a. It decreases stomach pH, allowing charged (ionized) drugs to be absorbed better.
  b. Grapefruit juice decreases absorption of plasma-bound drugs from both the stomach and intestines.
  c. It contains a compound that can inhibit intestinal cytochrome P-450, allowing more drug to be absorbed into the bloodstream.
  d. Drugs may be dissolved in grapefruit juice, allowing patients who can't swallow tablets to take their medication.

22. What statement is *true* about lipids?
  a. They are protein molecules.
  b. They generally attract water.
  c. They generally repel water.
  d. They are not part of the cell membrane.

23. Which route of administration does *not* require absorption?
  a. oral
  b. topical
  c. rectal
  d. intravenous
  e. transdermal

24. The rate at which a drug is eliminated from a specific volume of blood per unit of time is referred to as its
  a. duration of action.
  b. metabolism.
  c. clearance.
  d. distribution.

25. A physician might individualize a standard dosage in the case of a patient who is
  a. African American.
  b. malnourished.
  c. elderly.
  d. pregnant.
  e. All of the above

26. Some drugs may be administered by injection because they have substantial
  a. side effects.
  b. therapeutic effects.
  c. first-pass effects.
  d. ceiling effects.

27. How can the length of time required to achieve a drug's therapeutic level be shortened?
  a. accelerate the duration of action
  b. analyze a patient blood sample and adjust dosage accordingly
  c. vary doses and dosing intervals
  d. administer a loading dose

28. Drug tolerance would describe
  a. a person who uses cold tablets to manufacture methamphetamine.
  b. a patient on painkillers who needs an ever-increasing dose for relief.
  c. an alcoholic who craves beer, wine, or whiskey.
  d. a diabetic whose body cannot function without insulin.

29. What peroral route is administrated when a rapid action is desired?
  a. conjunctival
  b. aural
  c. buccal
  d. transdermal

30. What physiologic change frequently occurs in aging patients?
  a. auditory - hearing loss
  b. pulmonary - chronic obstructive pulmonary disease (COPD)
  c. cardiovascular - hypertension and coronary artery disease
  d. urinary - decreased number of functioning nephrons and incontinence
  e. All of the above

31. Which abbreviation should a prescriber use to indicate that a patient is to take the medication before meals?
  a. qd
  b. qh
  c. ud
  d. tid
  e. ac

32. What is the preferred dosage form for an antibiotic prescribed for a pediatric patient?
  a. intravenous solution
  b. tablet
  c. capsule
  d. oral solution
  e. suppository

33. What is a disadvantage of administering a drug by the peroral route?
  a. The drug generally takes longer to become effective.
  b. A professional healthcare worker must administer the drug.
  c. Administration can be painful and infection is possible.
  d. Drugs are always easily swallowed.
  e. It is the most expensive way to give medications.

34. When dispensing a new medication, the pharmacy technician should ask the patient,
  a. "Are your address and phone number current?"
  b. "Do you have health insurance?"
  c. "When is your birthday?"
  d. "Do you have any allergies?"
  e. All of the above

35. The result of decreased kidney elimination in the elderly causes an increased half life, which may require
  a. an increased dose
  b. changes in the drug form
  c. a decrease in the dose
  d. change in the pill size

36. Which immunization should the elderly who have had chicken pox have?
  a. zostavax (shingles)
  b. measles-mumps-rubella
  c. influenza
  d. diphtheria-tetanus-pertussis
  e. rotavirus

37. Poison ivy is the most common cause of
  a. allergic rhinitis.
  b. allergic dermatitis.
  c. contact dermatitis.
  d. urticaria.
  e. eczema.

38. What abbreviation should a pharmacy technician enter into the record if a patient has no allergies?
  a. nav
  b. NTA
  c. npo
  d. NKA

39. What is a critical role that technicians carry out?
  a. help ensure medication safety
  b. counsel patients on drug safety
  c. explain side effects to patients
  d. discuss medication schedules with patients

40. What patient information must pharmacy technicians handle?
  a. honoring an order to continue medication in patient transitions
  b. verifying addresses, dates of birth, and phone numbers of patients
  c. counseling patients
  d. making sure that tamper-resistant pads are used for oral prescriptions

Unit 2 Major Classes of Pharmaceutical Products I

Multiple Choice

Identify the choice that best completes the statement or answers the question.

1. Which of the following is an example of a gram-positive bacterium and an infection that it causes?
  a. *E. coli* resulting in urinary tract infections
  b. *Campylobacter* producing septicemia
  c. *Neisseria* resulting in gonorrhea
  d. *Treponema palladium* producing syphilis
  e. *Staphylococcus* resulting in toxic shock syndrome

2. What is true of a bacteriostatic antibiotic?
  a. It kills the invading organism.
  b. It is orally effective.
  c. It inhibits the growth or multiplication of bacteria.
  d. It is evenly distributed to both the host (patient) and the bacteria.
  e. It only affects gram-negative bacteria.

3. What bacterial pathway do sulfonamides interfere with?
  a. cell wall synthesis
  b. ribosome formation
  c. folic acid biosynthesis
  d. beta lactamase activity
  e. DNA replication

4. Which of the following drugs is associated with an adverse effect known as red man syndrome?
   a. amoxicillin (Amoxil, Trimox)
   b. vancomycin (Vancocin)
   c. chloramphenicol (Chloromycetin)
   d. metronidazole (Flagyl)
   e. clindamycin (Cleocin)
5. Disinfectants cannot be used systemically (internally) to treat infections because
   a. they are too costly.
   b. they would lose their specificity.
   c. they are effective only against gram-positive bacteria.
   d. they are not safe enough.
6. Sulfonamides are commonly used to treat
   a. venereal diseases.
   b. abscesses.
   c. heart valve infections.
   d. urinary tract infections.
   e. meningitis.
7. Which cephalosporins are most likely to react if a patient is allergic to penicillin?
   a. 1st generation
   b. 2nd generation
   c. 3rd generation
   d. 4th generation
   e. 5th generation
8. What is a mechanism of action of some antifungal drugs?
   a. prevent the synthesis of ribosomal proteins
   b. block the uptake of folic acid into the cell
   c. allow additional fluid to accumulate within the fungus, causing its cell wall to rupture
   d. interfere with the synthesis of ergosterol, a building block for fungal cell membranes
9. What is becoming a common dosing method for treating fungal nail infections?
   a. continuous dosing
   b. around-the-clock dosing
   c. daily dosing
   d. pulse dosing
10. Patients taking which of the following drugs should *not* drive at night?
    a. amphotericin B (Abelcet)
    b. fluconazole (Diflucan)
    c. voriconazole (VFEND)
    d. ketoconazole (Nizoral)
11. Which of the following antifungal drugs should be taken with a fatty meal and can be used safely in children?
    a. caspofungin (Cancidas)
    b. griseofulvin (Fulvicin P/G)
    c. clotrimazole (Mycelex-7)
    d. itraconazole (Sporanox)
    e. nystatin (Mycostatin)
12. What is an example of a chronic viral illness?
    a. influenza A
    b. influenza B
    c. common cold
    d. herpes
13. Which of the following antiviral drug is also effective in treating patients with parkinsonism?
    a. acyclovir (Zovirax)
    b. foscarnet (Foscavir)
    c. ribavirin (Capegus)
    d. amantadine (Symmetrel)
14. What class of drugs are used to treat varicella?
    a. antiretrovials
    b. pencillins
    c. antifungus agents
    d. antiviral agents
15. Which of the following choices represents a class of antiretroviral drugs?
    a. nucleoside reverse transcriptase inhibitor (NRTI)
    b. non-nucleoside reverse transcriptase inhibitor (NNRTI)
    c. protease inhibitor (PI)
    d. fusion inhibitor
    e. All of the above
16. The common cold is an example of a(n)
    a. generalized viral infection.
    b. chronic viral infection.
    c. systemic viral infection.
    d. fast viral infection.
    e. acute viral infection.

17. Which of the following drugs is a protease inhibitor?
    a. indinavir (Crixivan)
    b. delavirdine (Rescriptor)
    c. lamivudine (Epivir)
    d. tenofovir (Viread)
    e. stavudine (Zerit)

18. The primary PNS transmitters are
    a. dopamine and glutamate
    b. norepinephrine and glutamate
    c. norepinephrine and acetylcholine
    d. dopamine and norepinephrine

19. Manufacturers are reformulating combination narcotics that contain acetaminophen. The dose of acetaminophen they will all have will be
    a. 1 gram
    b. 750 mg
    c. 500 mg
    d. 325 mg

20. What property of nitrous oxide allows it to be used alone in dental procedures?
    a. It causes hypoxia.
    b. It induces analgesia only.
    c. Its effects are long lasting.
    d. It is a potent anesthetic.

21. Which narcotic is manufactured as a patch?
    a. fentanyl
    b. pentazocine
    c. Darvocet-N 100
    d. Dilaudid

22. Why are neuromuscular blocking agents an important adjunct to general anesthesia?
    a. They help to reverse benzodiazepine overdoses.
    b. They aid in the treatment of malignant hyperthermia.
    c. They are often used in ambulatory surgery.
    d. They facilitate endotracheal intubation.

23. What is the name for a short-acting class of local anesthetics?
    a. alkalines
    b. amides
    c. ethers
    d. esters

24. Which drug is used to treat opiate addiction?
    a. methohexital (Brevital)
    b. oxycodone (OxyContin)
    c. buprenorphine (Buprenex, Subutex)
    d. lorazepam (Ativan)
    e. neostigmine (Prostigmin)

25. Which migraine therapy is a controlled substance?
    a. almotriptan (Axert)
    b. dihydroergotamine (D.H.E. 45, Migranal)
    c. prochlorperazine (Reglan)
    d. butorphanol (Stadol, Stadol NS)

26. According to recent evidence, which drug used to treat migraine headaches has some potential for addiction?
    a. tramadol (Ultram)
    b. chlorpromazine (Thorazine)
    c. ketorolac (Toradol)
    d. prochlorperazine (Compazine)

27. Which two neurotransmitters are believed to be most involved with schizophrenia and the drugs used to treat this disorder?
    a. norepinephrine and serotonin
    b. dopamine and acetylcholine
    c. histamine and epinephrine
    d. dopamine and serotonin

28. Which drug used to treat sleep disorders is not a controlled substance?
    a. alprazolam (Xanax)
    b. zolpidem (Ambien)
    c. hydroxyzine (Vistaril)
    d. amobarbital (Amytal)

29. Which class of antidepressants is second-line therapy because of interactions with foods and other drugs?
    a. SSRIs
    b. TCAs
    c. MAOIs
    d. SNRIs

30. When does the first episode of bipolar disorder typically occur?
    a. about age 15
    b. about age 20
    c. about age 25
    d. about age 30

31. Drugs that are used to treat psychotic disorders
    a. reverse memory impairment, confusion, and intellectual deterioration.
    b. improve emotional and social withdrawal.
    c. reduce thought disorders, hallucinations, and delusions.
    d. a and b
    e. a, b, and c

32. Which of the following anticonvulsants is also used to treat manic episodes in bipolar mood disorders?
    a. valproic acid (Depakene)
    b. phenobarbital (Luminal)
    c. primidone (Mysoline)
    d. lithium (Lithobid)

33. The prevalence of Parkinson disease (parkinsonism) is highest in what age group?
    a. newborns
    b. adolescents
    c. mid 30s to 40s
    d. mid 40s to 50
    e. above age 60

34. What combination drug contains levodopa plus an inhibitor of peripheral levodopa metabolism?
    a. Sinemet
    b. Comtan
    c. Eldepryl
    d. Tasmar

35. Which drug used to treat ADD/ADHD is not a controlled substance?
    a. atomoxetine (Strattera)
    b. dexmethylphenidate (Focalin)
    c. methylphenidate (Ritalin)
    d. dextroamphetamine-amphetamine (Adderall)

36. Which drug listed below is used to treat patients with multiple sclerosis?
    a. interferon beta-1a (Avonex, Rebif)
    b. interferon beta-1b (Betaseron)
    c. mitoxantrone (Novantrone)
    d. baclofen (Lioresal)
    e. All of the above

37. What percentage of people with epilepsy have partial seizures?
    a. 45%
    b. 55%
    c. 65%
    d. 75%

38. A generalized seizure
    a. is the most common type of seizure.
    b. occurs in two distinct types.
    c. involves both hemispheres of the brain simultaneously.
    d. may progress to a partial seizure.

39. In the OROS system, what is the term for the part of a tablet that passes through the stool?
    a. specter tablet
    b. phantom tablet
    c. spirit tablet
    d. spook tablet
    e. ghost tablet

40. Methylphenidate, an agent used to treat children with ADD/ADHD, can best be characterized as a(n)
    a. sedative.
    b. stimulant.
    c. antidepressant.
    d. hypnotic.
    e. antianxiety agent.

41. What is a primary side effect of dextroamphetamine-amphetamine (Adderall)?
    a. bed-wetting in some children
    b. depression as the drug wears off
    c. weight gain and slow growth
    d. salivation
    e. nausea and vomiting

42. At the present time, drug therapy for multiple sclerosis seeks to
    a. relieve muscle spasticity.
    b. slow the progression of the disease.
    c. induce a calming effect.
    d. a and b
    e. a, b, and c

43. Which of the following is part of the profile for Alzheimer disease?
    a. seizures
    b. depression
    c. severe trembling
    d. loss of overall muscle control
    e. blindness

44. What drug that is used to treat Alzheimer disease is derived from daffodil bulbs?
    a. rivastigmine (Exelon)
    b. tacrine (Cognex)
    c. galamtamine (Razadyne)
    d. memantine (Namenda)

45. What class of drugs used to treat hypertension, angina, cardiac arrhythmias, and migraine headaches is contraindicated in asthma patients?
    a. antihistamines
    b. beta blockers
    c. ACE inhibitors
    d. calcium channel blockers

46. Which of the following antitussives is a DEA controlled substance?
    a. benzonatate (Tessalon)
    b. codeine
    c. dextromethorphan (Delsym)
    d. diphenhydramine (Benadryl)

47. What is the purpose of antitussives?
    a. to suppress dry and nonproductive coughs
    b. to relieve nasal congestion
    c. to rid the lungs and airway of mucus when coughing
    d. to relieve symptoms of allergies
    e. to alleviate vertigo

48. What are two types of receptors involved in the cough reflex?
    a. relaxed and spastic
    b. dilated and constricted
    c. smooth and striped
    d. stretch and irritant

49. What is rhinitis medicamentosa?
    a. rebound phenomenon
    b. nasal edema
    c. rebound receptor sensitivity
    d. b and c
    e. All of the above

50. Why do pharmacies in many areas of the country currently limit the sale of pseudoephedrine (Sudafed)?
    a. Pseudoephedrine is a different name for ephedrine.
    b. Pseudoephedrine is in short supply.
    c. Pseudoephedrine has abuse potential.
    d. Pseudoephedrine has many adverse side effects.
    e. Pseudoephedrine has questionable efficacy.

Unit 3 Major Classes of Pharmaceutical Products II

Multiple Choice

Identify the choice that best completes the statement or answers the question.

1. What is the most common cause of drug-induced ulcers?
    a. caffeine
    b. aspirin
    c. alcohol
    d. iron

2. What GI disorder is characterized by inflammation of the large bowel with the patient experiencing diarrhea containing blood, mucus, and pus?
    a. ulcerative colitis
    b. gastritis
    c. gastroesophageal reflux disease (GERD)
    d. malabsorption syndrome

3. Patients on long-term narcotic pain medication should also be taking a(n)
    a. osmotic laxative.
    b. saline laxative.
    c. stimulant laxative.
    d. antiflatulent.
    e. bowel evacuant.

4. The sensation of the room spinning when one gets up or changes positions is known as
    a. hyperuricemia.
    b. paralytic ileus.
    c. gastric stasis.
    d. vertigo.
    e. alopecia.

5. Pyrantel (Pin X) treats pinworms by
   a. increasing permeability of worm cells
   b. binding to tubular proteins
   c. paralyzing the worm
   d. blocking energy production
6. What do the kidneys regulate?
   a. blood plasma volume
   b. concentration of waste products in the blood
   c. electrolyte concentrations
   d. plasma acid-base balance
   e. All of the above
7. Which of the following drugs may be used to prevent rejection in kidney transplant patients?
   a. epoetin alfa (Epogen, Procrit)
   b. cyclosporine (Sandimmune)
   c. oxybutynin (Ditropan)
   d. tolterodine (Detrol)
8. When taking which of the following antibiotics (or combinations) should sunscreen be used?
   a. amoxicillin-clavulanate (Augmentin)
   b. sulfamethoxazole-trimethoprim (Bactrim, Cotrim, Septra)
   c. ciprofloxacin (Cipro)
   d. a and c
   e. b and c
9. How does Toviaz (fesoterodine) prevent bladder leaks?
   a. blocks cholinergic receptors
   b. prevents bladder from squeezing
   c. stimulates cholinergic receptors
   d. contracts sphincter
10. What might be a sign of stage 2 renal disease?
    a. anorexia
    b. nocturia
    c. pruritus
    d. metabolic acidosis
    e. hypocalcemia
11. Which of the following is a laboratory test of kidney function?
    a. hemoglobin
    b. blood glucose
    c. serum creatinine
    d. HDL/LDL
    e. A1C
12. Which is not a symptom of overactive bladder?
    a. urgency
    b. frequency
    c. incontinence
    d. infection
13. What is the purpose of diuretics?
    a. to relieve painful urination
    b. to increase urine output
    c. to treat urinary tract infections
    d. to shrink the bladder
    e. to decrease urine output
14. Which class of diuretics should be prescribed with caution to patients on ACE inhibitors?
    a. thiazides
    b. loops
    c. potassium-sparing
    d. carbonic anhydrase inhibitors
    e. osmotics
15. Patients on diuretics frequently need what supplement?
    a. vitamin D
    b. magnesium
    c. calcium
    d. potassium
    e. all of the above
16. Which of the following drug classes is *not* used to treat angina?
    a. nitrates
    b. beta blockers
    c. calcium channel blockers
    d. angiotensin II receptor antagonists
17. What antiarrhythmic agent is also an anticonvulsant agent?
    a. dofetilide (Tikosyn)
    b. procainamide (Procanbid, Pronestyl)
    c. digoxin (Lanoxicaps, Lanoxin)
    d. phenytoin (Dilantin)

18. Which of the following anticoagulant drugs is available in tablet form?
   a. heparin
   b. bivalirudin (Angiomax)
   c. dalteparin (Fragmin)
   d. warfarin (Coumadin)

19. What is *not* characteristic of cholesterol?
   a. It is a waxlike, powdery substance.
   b. It is an odorless, white substance.
   c. It is in foods of animal origin.
   d. It is in foods of plant origin.

20. What is the staging of a patient whose blood pressure is consistently 140–159/90–99 mm Hg?
   a. normal
   b. prehypertension
   c. hypertension stage 1
   d. hypertension stage 2
   e. posthypertension

21. Which class of drugs is used to treat angina, arrhythmia, hypertension, and myocardial infarction?
   a. ACE inhibitors
   b. beta blockers
   c. calcium channel blockers
   d. vasodilators

22. The lethal dose of aspirin for an adult is usually more than
   a. 650 mg.
   b. 1 g.
   c. 3.5 g.
   d. 10 g.

23. What clinical effect or side effect of aspirin is also produced by acetaminophen (Tylenol)?
   a. fever reduction
   b. GI irritation
   c. altered platelet adhesion and bleeding
   d. inflammation reduction

24. NSAIDs can interact with which of the following drug classes?
   a. antibiotics
   b. beta adrenergic agonists
   c. oral hypoglycemics
   d. antacids

25. What warning label should appear on prescriptions for muscle relaxants?
   a. May cause drowsiness.
   b. This drug interferes with the effectiveness of oral contraceptives.
   c. Do not take if pregnant.
   d. Refrigerate after opening.
   e. May turn urine blue.

26. What is an example of somatic pain?
   a. appendicitis attack
   b. backache
   c. kidney stones
   d. migraine headache
   e. gastritis

27. In addition to providing primary drug therapy for arthritis, NSAIDs are commonly used to treat
   a. heartburn.
   b. diarrhea.
   c. menstrual cramps.
   d. nausea and vomiting.
   e. high blood pressure.

28. Which of the following drugs or drug classes may cause male impotence?
   a. alcohol
   b. corticosteroids
   c. haloperidol (Haldol)
   d. opiates
   e. All of the above

29. What is a danger of using nicotine in combination with estrogen?
   a. birth defects
   b. ineffective birth control
   c. increased risk of blood clots
   d. increased risk of breast cancer
   e. All of the above

30. What oral contraceptive may cause weight loss in patients?
   a. ethinyl estradiol-drospirenone (Yasmine, Yaz)
   b. ethinyl estradiol-etonogestrel (NuvaRing)
   c. estradiol-drospirenone (Angeliq)
   d. estradiol cypionate-medroxyprogesterone (Lunelle)

31. Which of the following drugs acts to prevent bone loss by modulating estrogen receptors?
   a. alendronate (Fosamax)
   b. risedronate (Actonel)
   c. zoledronic acid (Zometa)
   d. raloxifene (Evista)
   e. teriparatide (Forteo)

32. Approximately what percentage of persons older than 60 years have diabetes?
   a. 5%
   b. 10%
   c. 15%
   d. 20%
   e. 25%

33. Which of the following oral hypoglycemic agents acts by interfering with carbohydrate metabolism and glucose absorption?
   a. acarbose (Precose)
   b. pioglitazone (Actos)
   c. glipizide (Glucotrol)
   d. metformin (Glucophage)

34. Which of the following is a characteristic of hyperthyroidism?
   a. thick tongue
   b. protruding eyeballs
   c. short stature
   d. mental retardation
   e. swollen eyelids

35. Which hormone, released by the hypothalamic-pituitary axis, stimulates the ovaries to produce estrogen?
   a. FSH
   b. ACTH
   c. ADH
   d. LH
   e. GnRH

36. What is a symptom of estrogen deficiency?
   a. vasomotor instability
   b. dyspareunia
   c. atrophic vulvovaginitis
   d. a and b
   e. a, b, and c

37. Hormone replacement therapy is controversial because it is associated with increased risk of
   a. osteoporosis.
   b. cardiovascular disease.
   c. breast cancer.
   d. memory loss.
   e. All of the above

38. What is the major reason to use corticosteroids?
   a. to prevent bone loss
   b. to reduce inflammation
   c. to open airways
   d. to reduce symptoms of menopause
   e. to build muscle

39. Growth hormone
   a. increases the rate of protein synthesis.
   b. stimulates the growth of muscle and connective tissue.
   c. increases the rate of glucose use.
   d. a and b
   e. a, b, and c

40. Which drug used to treat head lice is extracted from chrysanthemum seeds?
   a. Tinactin (Tolnaftate)
   b. lindane
   c. Nix (permethrin)
   d. Rid (Pyrethin)

41. Which of the following drugs is used to treat acne vulgaris?
   a. tretinoin (Retin-A)
   b. botulinum toxin type A (Botox)
   c. alefacept (Amevive)
   d. nystatin (Mycostatin)

42. Which of the following drugs is a neurotoxin used to treat facial wrinkles?
   a. botulinum toxin type A (Botox)
   b. pimecrolimus (Elidel)
   c. azelaic acid (Azelex)
   d. tretinoin (Retin-A)

43. Which substance inhibits growth and development of microorganisms but does not necessarily kill them?
   a. antiseptic
   b. disinfectant
   c. fungicide
   d. germicide

44. What causes age-related macular degeneration (AMD)?
   a. excessive sun exposure
   b. adverse reaction to antibiotics
   c. infection
   d. unknown

45. What is the most commonly occurring eye disease?
   a. conjunctivitis (dry eye)
   b. cataracts
   c. glaucoma
   d. CMV retinitis

46. Another name for pink eye is
   a. macular degeneration
   b. conjunctivitis
   c. glaucoma
   d. dry eye

47. Ringworm is a skin disorder caused by a
   a. parasite.
   b. protozoan.
   c. fungus.
   d. bacterium.
   e. head louse.

48. Topical corticosteroids should be applied as a thin film and used sparingly because
   a. they can have an intense drying effect.
   b. they can metabolize in the GI tract.
   c. they can cause photosensitivity.
   d. they can penetrate the skin.
   e. they can produce a state of denervation.

49. What is the term for an infestation of lice?
   a. petechiae
   b. pediculosis
   c. psoriasis
   d. pellagra
   e. prostatitis

50. The pharmacy technician should inform the pharmacist if
   a. the physician prescribes eardrops for an eye infection.
   b. the physician prescribes an otic antibiotic but not an accompanying pain reliever.
   c. the physician prescribes an otic solution for a patient with a tube in the ear.
   d. a and b
   e. a, b, and c

Unit 4 Chemotherapy and Miscellaneous Pharmaceutical Products

Multiple Choice

Identify the choice that best completes the statement or answers the question.

1. The protein that is extracted from pooled resources of human plasma or tissues
   a. is available in small quantities.
   b. is available in large quantities.
   c. comes from unlimited sources.
   d. has no risk of viral contamination.

2. Which drug is *not* used to treat leukemia?
   a. bicalutamide (Casodex)
   b. daunorubicin (Cerubidine)
   c. doxorubicin (Adriamycin)
   d. fludarbine (Fludara)

3. Which of the following statements about erythropoietin is true?
   a. It is produced by the kidneys.
   b. The recombinant DNA product is known as epoetin alfa (Epogen, Procrit).
   c. Erythropoietin increases the production of red blood cells.
   d. The drug should not be shaken, as this may denature the glycoprotein and inactivate it.
   e. All of the above

4. What is the most common immunoglobulin, making up about 80% of the total in plasma?
   a. IgA
   b. IgD
   c. IgE
   d. IgG
   e. IgM

5. Before receiving most chemotherapy medication, patients must be pre-medicated to alleviate the side effects. Which drug would not be used for this purpose?
   a. diphenhydramine (Benadryl)
   b. acetaminophen (Tylenol)
   c. ondansetron (Zofran)
   d. ibuprofen (Motrin, Advil)
   e. epirubicin (Ellence)

6. Which of the following hormones is *incorrectly* paired with the type of cancer it is used to treat?
   a. abarelix (Plenaxis) - prostate
   b. flutamide (Eulexin) - breast
   c. triptorelin (Trelstar) - prostate
   d. megestrol - breast

7. Which drug listed below is indicated for ovarian cancer, should not be used in pregnant patients, and almost always causes hair loss?
   a. paclitaxel (Taxol)
   b. cisplatin (Platinol)
   c. fludarabine (Fludara)
   d. chlorambucil (Leukeran)

8. What drug is used to treat Hodgkin disease?
   a. imatinib (Gleevec)
   b. gefitnib (Iressa)
   c. pemetrexad (Alimta)
   d. procarbazine (Matulane)

9. What drug combination is known as "Magic Swizzle"?
   a. phenol-sodium borate-sodium bicarbonate-glycerin
   b. chlorhexidine gluconate
   c. lidocaine-diphenhydramine-Maalox
   d. phenol-sodium borate-sodium bicarbonate-glycerin

10. For what drug has the National Cancer Institute recommended that oncologists prescribe it to patients for no more than 5 years?
    a. tamoxifen (Nolvadex)
    b. anastrozole (Arimidex)
    c. fulvestrant (Faslodex)
    d. letrozole (Femara)
    e. All of the above

11. The final step in the natural process for making proteins is
    a. copying.
    b. transcription.
    c. replication.
    d. translation.

12. Which class of recombinant DNA drugs is used to influence the bone marrow to produce blood cells?
    a. colony-stimulating factor
    b. biologic-response modifier
    c. fibrinolytic agent
    d. secretion-thinning enzyme
    e. hematologic agent

13. What are immunoglobulins?
    a. substances that mediate an inflammatory reaction
    b. molecules not bound to an antigen
    c. substances that are foreign to the body
    d. proteins with antibody activity

14. Which immunoglobulin is the main Ig in salivary and bronchial secretions?
    a. IgG
    b. IgM
    c. IgA
    d. IgE
    e. IgD

15. Which organ is *not* part of the lymphatic system?
    a. tonsils
    b. pancreas
    c. thymus
    d. spleen
    e. They are all part of the lymphatic system.

16. Many cancer patients have oral complications; which drug would not be used to treat this problem?
    a. cevimeline (Evoxac)
    b. folinic acid (Leucovorin)
    c. chlorhexadine (Peridex)
    d. pilocarpine (Salagen)

17. Neoplastic disease occurs when
    a. there is controlled cellular growth.
    b. normal cellular growth control mechanisms become altered.
    c. there is a bacterial infection.
    d. there is a viral infection.

18. Antitumor drugs are
    a. most efficient when tumor cells are dividing rapidly.
    b. extremely toxic.
    c. periodically stopped for two to six weeks.
    d. a and c
    e. a, b, and c

19. A cytoprotective agent is also known as a(n)
    a. antirejection drug.
    b. cholinergic agent.
    c. biological-response modifier.
    d. rescue agent.

20. Which of the following is *not* a drug that is used to prevent mucositis resulting from chemotherapy?
    a. pilocarpine (Salagen)
    b. hydrogen peroxide (Peroxyl)
    c. meperidine (Demerol)
    d. cevimeline (Evoxac)
    e. chlorhexidine gluconate (Peridex)

21. Drugs for the prevention of breast cancer recurrence attempt to intercept the production of
    a. estrone.
    b. estrogen.
    c. progesterone.
    d. medroxyprogesterone.
    e. norethindrone.

22. Which of the following is a water-soluble vitamin?
    a. vitamin A
    b. vitamin C
    c. vitamin D3
    d. vitamin E
    e. All of the above

23. Which antidote is used for an overdose of acetaminophen?
    a. acetylcysteine
    b. atropine
    c. glucagon
    d. fomepizole

24. What is osteomalacia?
    a. demineralization and weakening of the bones
    b. instability of cell membranes
    c. dark red coloration on skin exposed to air and light
    d. onset of dementia

25. What term describes a method in which the patient is fed through a vein?
    a. enteral nutrition
    b. total parenteral nutrition
    c. peroral nutrition
    d. None of the above

26. What is a complication associated with parenteral nutrition?
    a. acid-base imbalance
    b. high serum lipid concentrations
    c. electrolyte imbalance
    d. liver toxicity
    e. All of the above

27. Which dietary supplement is *incorrectly* paired with its medicinal use?
    a. echinacea - common cold
    b. chondroitin/glucosamine - arthritis
    c. melatonin - sleep
    d. garlic - impotence

28. The primary cation of intracellular fluid is
    a. sodium
    b. potassium
    c. calcium
    d. magnesium

29. What toxin with the potential for bioterrorism is derived from the castor bean?
    a. atropine
    b. botulin
    c. tuberemia
    d. anthrax
    e. ricin

30. Alcoholics are often deficient in
    a. vitamin B_1.
    b. vitamin B_9.
    c. vitamin B_{12}.
    d. a and b
    e. a, b, and c

31. Proportionally, who has the highest amount of body water?
    a. a lean, well-muscled male adult
    b. an obese adult
    c. an adult female
    d. an elderly person
    e. a newborn

32. Which of the following blood pH levels indicates acidosis?
    a. 7.47
    b. 7.41
    c. 7.38
    d. 7.33

33. In contrast to two-in-ones, three-in-one TPN solutions
    a. are more stable and thus last longer.
    b. allow precipitants to be easily seen.
    c. may crack or separate.
    d. can remain at room temperature for 48 hours.

34. Which of the following appears on a label for an herbal product?
    a. proven medical uses
    b. contents
    c. drug interactions
    d. potential side effects
    e. All of the above

35. Which of the following is the leading cause of fatal poisonings in children?
    a. mouthwash
    b. antidepressants
    c. iron tablets
    d. aspirin

36. What is the most common route for poisoning?
    a. injection
    b. skin contamination
    c. inhalation
    d. ingestion

37. Once a person has ingested poison, what are the primary concerns?
    a. eliminating it
    b. diminishing the effects
    c. interactions
    d. a and b
    e. All of the above

38. Which of the following is the primary agent for gastric lavage in an emergency room?
    a. cathartics
    b. sorbitol
    c. activated charcoal
    d. magnesium sulfate
    e. All of the above

39. What is the pharmacy technician's responsibility when a Blue Alert cart is returned to the pharmacy?
    a. Restock drugs.
    b. Remove and replace expired drugs.
    c. Remove and replace drugs that will expire in the next month.
    d. a and b
    e. a, b, and c

40. What are the three forms of plague?
    a. septicemic, inhalation, and ingestion
    b. bubonic, septicemic, and pneumonic
    c. cutaneous, inhalation, and gastrointestinal
    d. bubonic, cutaneous, and inhalation

Midterm Exam 1

Questions from this exam cover Units 1 and 2 (chapters 1 – 9)

Multiple Choice

Identify the choice that best completes the statement or answers the question.

1. How are legend drugs sold in the United States?
    a. with the label "Caution: Federal law prohibits dispensing without prescription"
    b. with the label "Legend drugs may not be refilled by phone"
    c. either by prescription or over the counter
    d. with clear warnings about their abuse potential

2. Into how many schedules are controlled substances categorized in the United States?
    a. 2
    b. 3
    c. 4
    d. 5
    e. 6

3. What is a medication guide?
    a. a list of drugs that must be monitored for elderly patients
    b. protection against disease
    c. a script issued in an institutional setting
    d. the part of the script that provides directives
    e. specific information about certain types of drugs that is required by the FDA to be made available to the patient

4. Alternative medicines, including herbs, supplements, and homeopathic remedies
    a. have been tested and approved by the FDA.
    b. should not be taken by patients.
    c. are bioequivalent from manufacturer to manufacturer.
    d. can interact adversely with prescription drugs.
    e. All of the above

5. What term is used to describe a drug that binds to a receptor and has an action similar to that of an endogenous chemical?
    a. agonist
    b. antagonist
    c. antidote
    d. inducer
    e. dose

6. In what way are the capillaries in the central nervous system (CNS) different from other capillaries?
    a. They contain double membranes, making it more difficult for lipid-soluble drugs to enter the CNS.
    b. They lack essential drug transporters necessary to distribute drugs into the CNS.
    c. They are enveloped by glial cells, which are additional barriers against water-soluble compounds.
    d. Except for sedatives and analgesics, the meninges must be disturbed before other drugs can enter the CNS.

7. What statement is *true* about lipids?
    a. They are protein molecules.
    b. They generally attract water.
    c. They generally repel water.
    d. They are not part of the cell membrane.

8. What is the advantage of metabolizing drugs to more water-soluble forms?
    a. Water-soluble forms can more readily be passed through cell membranes.
    b. Water-soluble forms can more readily be excreted by the liver.
    c. Water-soluble forms can increase the rate of gastric emptying.
    d. Water-soluble forms can pass through the blood-brain barrier.
    e. Water-soluble forms can decrease the amount of drug lost to protein binding.

9. A person on calcium for osteoporosis also needs to take vitamin D. Without vitamin D, the calcium cannot get into the bone. The relationship between calcium and vitamin D is an example of
    a. addition.
    b. antagonism.
    c. potentiation.
    d. synergism.

10. What is the correct form to express that a drug should be taken "every day"?
    a. PO
    b. q week
    c. DAW
    d. prn
    e. To prevent confusion, it is recommended that this term not be abbreviated.

11. What abbreviation should be used if a prescriber wants a drug to be administered immediately?
    a. ac
    b. hr
    c. stat
    d. qid
    e. npo

12. Which are the rights for correct drug administration?
    a. right patient
    b. right drug
    c. right strength
    d. right time
    e. alll of the above

13. How are many vaccines stored?
    a. in dark rooms
    b. in syringes
    c. at refrigerated temperatures
    d. at room temperatures

14. Medication reconciliation is
    a. providing a complete and accurate drug profile to each health care provider who cares for a patient
    b. the process of allowing the prescriber's computer system to talk to the pharmacy's computer system
    c. specific information about certain types of drugs
    d. information printed on a drug package to alert prescribers to potential problems
    e. a method of describing the process of absorption
15. What does the term *mortality* mean?
    a. rate of death from a particular disease
    b. rate of occurrence of a diseased state or condition
    c. exposure to an inactivated part of an infectious organism
    d. concentration of an antibody in the bloodstream
16. Bacteria that require oxygen to survive are known as
    a. aerobic.
    b. anaerobic.
    c. nosocomial.
    d. gram-positive.
    e. antibiotics.
17. What are two general signs that an infection is bacterial in origin?
    a. fever above 98.6 degrees Fahrenheit and runny nose
    b. blood in sputum and chills
    c. aches and fever (above 100.2 degrees Fahrenheit)
    d. white blood cell count above 12,000 and fever above 101 degrees Fahrenheit
18. What is the biggest challenge in developing a new antibiotic?
    a. keeping the cost as low as possible
    b. finding a way to make the drug water soluble
    c. killing the bacteria without harming the patient
    d. assuring distribution to all tissues in the body including heart, brain, and muscle
    e. making sure it is bactericidal
19. Synercid (quinupristin/dalfopristin) is an antibiotic belonging to which drug class?
    a. penicillins
    b. streptogammins
    c. macrolides
    d. quinolones
20. What percentage of patients allergic to penicillins are also allergic to cephalosporins?
    a. 1%
    b. 5%
    c. 10%
    d. 20%
    e. 25%
21. To minimize GI upset some drugs must be taken
    a. in the morning
    b. in smaller doses
    c. once daily
    d. with food
    e. at bedtime
22. What can the technician do to make a big difference in compliance in the pediatric population?
    a. flavor the drug
    b. color the drug
    c. put the drug in a funny bottle
    d. warm the drug
    e. cool the drug
23. What is a common target of fungal infections?
    a. brain
    b. heart
    c. lungs
    d. ears
    e. nails
24. Which latent virus can reappear in response to menstruation?
    a. histoplasmosis
    b. candida
    c. varicella
    d. genital herpes

25. What is another name for an individual virus particle?
    a. capsid
    b. virion
    c. naked virus
    d. interferon

26. Which of the following choices represents a class of antiretroviral drugs?
    a. nucleoside reverse transcriptase inhibitor (NRTI)
    b. non-nucleoside reverse transcriptase inhibitor (NNRTI)
    c. protease inhibitor (PI)
    d. fusion inhibitor
    e. All of the above

27. Which drug class can precipitate a fungal infection?
    a. diuretics
    b. ace inhibitors
    c. NSAIDS
    d. antibiotics
    e. narcotics

28. Why are most potent anesthetics gases or vapors?
    a. Gases or vapors can be used for general or local anesthesia.
    b. Gases or vapors are more easily controlled.
    c. Gases or vapors provide more pain relief than other forms of anesthesia.
    d. Gases or vapors eliminate the patient's memory of the procedure.

29. Which of the following are classified as antiemetic agents?
    a. Phenergan
    b. Reglan
    c. Compazine
    d. a and b
    e. All of the above

30. Which of the following drugs is classified as a tricyclic antidepressant and has significant anticholinergic side effects?
    a. lithium (Eskalith)
    b. imipramine (Tofranil)
    c. fluoxetine (Prozac)
    d. venlafaxine (Effexor)

31. Which drugs listed below are used to treat narcolepsy?
    a. Xanax (alprazolam) and Tranxene (clorazepate)
    b. Vistaril (hydroxyzine) and Provigil (modafinil)
    c. Nuvagil (armodafinil) and Provigil (modafinil)
    d. Ambien (zolpidem) and Nuvigil (armodafinil)

32. Duration of sleep medications should be limited to:
    a. no limit on duration
    b. 1 year
    c. 4 to 6 weeks
    d. 6 months

33. Which drug is not a benzodiazepine?
    a. Restoril (temazepam)
    b. Valium (diazepam)
    c. Ambien (zolpidem)
    d. Dalmane (flurazepam)
    e. Tranxene (clorazepate)

34. Low doses of prochlorperazine (Compazine) are commonly used for
    a. diarrhea.
    b. constipation.
    c. nausea and vomiting.
    d. menstrual cramps.
    e. severe headaches.

35. Which drug is not an alcohol antagonist?
    a. Campral (alcamprosate)
    b. Antabuse (disulfiram)
    c. ReVia (naltrexone)
    d. Valium (diazepam)

36. Which of the following anticonvulsants is also used to treat manic episodes in bipolar mood disorders?
    a. valproic acid (Depakene)
    b. phenobarbital (Luminal)
    c. primidone (Mysoline)
    d. lithium (Lithobid)

37. Which two neurotransmitters are out of balance in Parkinson disease?
    a. serotonin and dopamine
    b. dopamine and acetylcholine
    c. acetylcholine and serotonin
    d. epinephrine and dopamine

38. What dopamine precursor is used to treat Parkinson patients?
    a. amantadine (Symmetrel)
    b. bromocriptine (Parlodel)
    c. benztropine (Cogentin)
    d. levodopa (Dopar)
39. What class of drugs may be used to diagnose and treat myasthenia gravis?
    a. neuromuscular blockers
    b. acetylcholinesterase inhibitors
    c. dopamine (D1) antagonists
    d. muscarinic receptor antagonists
40. Which drug used to treat ADD/ADHD is not a controlled substance?
    a. clonidine (Catapres)
    b. dexmethylphenidate (Focalin)
    c. methylphenidate (Ritalin)
    d. dextroamphetamine-amphetamine (Adderall)
41. Why might a prescribing physician prefer donepezil (Aricept) over tacrine (Cognex) for Alzheimer disease?
    a. Donepezil is given once a day.
    b. Donepezil does not result in nausea, vomiting, and diarrhea.
    c. Donepezil improves memory and alertness.
    d. none of the above
    e. a, b, and c
42. Which herb might be used to treat Alzheimer's Disease?
    a. garlic
    b. ginger
    c. ginkgo
    d. ginseng
43. Which of the following is a potentially life-threatening condition in which the patient has difficulty breathing, has blue lips and nail beds, may lose consciousness, and does not respond to normal management?
    a. status emphysema
    b. chronic bronchitis
    c. status asthmaticus
    d. acute bronchitis
44. With which device, used to administer asthma or COPD medications, does a stream of air flow past a liquid to create a fine mist for the patient to inhale?
    a. metered dose inhaler
    b. spacer
    c. nebulizer
    d. peak flow meter
45. Which inhaler would be used as a rescue inhaler?
    a. levalbuterol (Xopenex)
    b. tiotropium (Spiriva)
    c. salmeterol (Serevent)
    d. albuterol (Pro-Air)
    e. fluticasone (Flonase, Flovent)
46. What role can pharmacy technicians play in asthma drug therapy?
    a. They can be alert to patient overdependence on short-acting beta-2 agonists.
    b. They can explain how to take an asthma drug.
    c. They can suggest which asthma drug to take.
    d. a and b
47. What is the best way for a patient with bronchitis to break up mucus and cough up secretions?
    a. take cough syrup
    b. use a mucolytic
    c. drink lots of water
    d. use a nebulizer
    e. tap on the lungs
48. Cystic fibrosis is a pulmonary disease that also involves the
    a. cardiovascular system.
    b. gastrointestinal system.
    c. nervous system.
    d. excretory system.
    e. skeletal system.
49. Which drug is an expectorant?
    a. pseudoephedrine
    b. phenylephrine
    c. guaifenesin
    d. genzonataate
    e. diphenhydramine

50. Almost every OTC sleeping pill contains
    a. diphenhydramine
    b. desloratadine
    c. cetrizine
    d. loratadine

Midterm Exam II

Questions from this exam cover Units 3 and 4 (chapters 10 - 17)

Multiple Choice

Identify the choice that best completes the statement or answers the question.

1. What is a potential problem associated with low-fiber diets?
    a. constipation
    b. diarrhea
    c. gastritis
    d. GERD

2. Which drug below is approved for chronic idiopathic constipation?
    a. lubiprostone (Amitiza)
    b. hydrocortisone (Anusol HC)
    c. metoclopramide (Reglan)
    d. granisetron (Kytril)
    e. ondansetron (Zofran)

3. What drug has been used since the seventeenth century and is now used in combination with other drugs to treat malaria?
    a. quinine (Qualaquin)
    b. mefloquine (Lariam)
    c. doxycycline (Vibramycin)
    d. chloroquine (Aralen)

4. Which of the following is used as phase I medication to treat GERD?
    a. proton pump inhibitors
    b. antacids
    c. coating agents
    d. cholinergic agents
    e. H_2 receptor antagonists

5. Antimotility medications are used to treat
    a. chronic diarrhea.
    b. short-term constipation.
    c. acute malabsorption.
    d. terminal gastritis.

6. Psyllium (Fiberall, Metamucil) is used as a(n)
    a. laxative.
    b. antidiarrheal.
    c. cholesterol-lowering agent.
    d. a and b
    e. a, b, and c

7. What form of hepatitis is most commonly spread through blood transfusions or illicit drug use?
    a. hepatitis A
    b. acute hepatitis B
    c. chronic hepatitis B
    d. hepatitis C

8. Which of the following damages the kidney?
    a. damage to the vascular tree
    b. change in glomerular permeability
    c. autoimmune reactions
    d. radiocontrast dyes
    e. all of the above

9. Which of the following drugs is not used to prevent rejection in kidney transplant patients?
    a. cyclosporine (Sandimmune)
    b. epoetin alfa (Epogen, Procrit)
    c. mycophenolate (Cellcept)
    d. mycophenolate (Myfortic)

10. __________ is the only oral therapy for interstitial cystitis (inflammation of the urinary bladder).
    a. bethanechol (Urechholine)
    b. duloxetine (Cymbalta)
    c. pentosan polysulfate sodium (Elmiron)
    d. toltorodine (Detrol)
    e. trospium (Santura)

11. What is the function of the ureter?
    a. to regulate the concentration of waste products in urine
    b. to conduct urine from the kidneys to the bladder
    c. to exchange potassium in the urine for sodium
    d. to collect urine until it is released from the body
    e. to conduct urine from the bladder to outside of the body

12. Which of the following is a laboratory test of kidney function?
   a. hemoglobin
   b. blood glucose
   c. serum creatinine
   d. HDL/LDL
   e. A1C

13. What is the most common side effect of iron sucrose (Venofer)?
   a. hypotension
   b. fatigue
   c. diarrhea
   d. headaches

14. What antibiotic used to treat UTIs may turn urine brown or dark yellow?
   a. amoxicillin (Amoxil)
   b. phenazopyridine (Azo-Standard, Uristat)
   c. ampicillin (Principen)
   d. nitrofursantoin (Macrobid, Macrodantin)

15. Why should TCAs, anticholinergics, oral bronchodilators, and certain other drugs *not* be used for patients with BPH?
   a. They cause hypertension.
   b. They affect bladder function.
   c. They hinder sexual performance.
   d. They cause headaches and dizziness.

16. Which class of drugs used to treat renal problems is also used to lower blood pressure?
   a. antibiotics
   b. antivirals
   c. diuretics
   d. antifungals
   e. calcium channel blockers

17. What form of angina is characterized by coronary artery spasm?
   a. stable angina
   b. unstable angina
   c. variant angina
   d. coronaspasm

18. Which of the following drugs used for MIs and stroke prevention blocks ADP receptors, reducing platelet adhesion and aggregation?
   a. aspirin
   b. clopidogrel (Plavix)
   c. pentoxifylline (Trental)
   d. dipyridamole (Persantine)

19. What class of drugs that is used to dissolve clots must be reconstituted in water and then gently swirled, never shaken?
   a. anticoagulants
   b. antiplatelets
   c. fibrinolytic agents
   d. glycoprotein antagonists

20. Which of the following drugs reduces cholesterol levels by inhibiting HMG-CoA reductase, the enzyme that catalyzes the rate-limiting step in the synthesis of cholesterol?
   a. gemfibrozil (Lopid)
   b. simvastatin (Zocor)
   c. niacin (Simcor)
   d. ezetimibe (Zetia)

21. Diuretics help to lower blood pressure by
   a. reducing preload.
   b. increasing preload.
   c. reducing afterload.
   d. increasing afterload.

22. Patients with hyperlipidemia should avoid
   a. estrogen.
   b. calcium channel blockers.
   c. loop diuretics.
   d. clonidine.

23. Which of the following is true about skeletal muscles?
   a. voluntarily controlled
   b. involuntarily controlled
   c. smooth texture
   d. cordlike

24. How do salicylates reduce fever?
   a. increasing blood flow to skin and inhibiting PG synthesis
   b. decreasing blood flow to skin and inhibiting PG synthesis
   c. increasing blood flow to hypothalamus
   d. decreasing blood flow to hypothalamus

25. Which of the following is an example of a disease-modifying antirheumatic drug (DMARD)?
   a. adalimunab (Humira)
   b. anakinra (Kineret)
   c. methotrexate (Rheumatrex)
   d. azathioprine (Imuran)
   e. All of the above

26. In addition to providing primary drug therapy for arthritis, NSAIDs are commonly used to treat
   a. heartburn.
   b. diarrhea.
   c. menstrual cramps.
   d. nausea and vomiting.
   e. high blood pressure.

27. What causes gouty arthritis?
   a. improper excretion of uric acid
   b. long-term elevated LDL cholesterol levels
   c. chronic hypertension
   d. abnormal activity by chondrocytes, or cartilage cells

28. Which of the following drugs acts to prevent bone loss by modulating estrogen receptors?
   a. alendronate (Fosamax)
   b. risedronate (Actonel)
   c. zoledronic acid (Zometa)
   d. raloxifene (Evista)
   e. teriparatide (Forteo)

29. Which of the following is a characteristic of hyperthyroidism?
   a. thick tongue
   b. protruding eyeballs
   c. short stature
   d. mental retardation
   e. swollen eyelids

30. Hormone replacement therapy is controversial because it is associated with increased risk of
   a. osteoporosis.
   b. cardiovascular disease.
   c. breast cancer.
   d. memory loss.
   e. All of the above

31. Acute hypoglycemia occurs when
   a. plasma glucose is above 600 mg/dL of blood.
   b. blood glucose levels two hours after eating are 200–400 mg/dL.
   c. fasting glucose is 80–120 mg/dL of blood.
   d. blood glucose levels fall below 70 mg/dL.

32. What features are characteristic of rosacea?
   a. redness, warmth, local pain, and plaque
   b. flushing, erythema, papules, and pustules
   c. red, scaly skin and arthritis
   d. erythema, edema, and vesicles

33. With which of the following drugs could an antibiotic interfere?
   a. benzodiazepines
   b. oral contraceptives
   c. topicals
   d. anesthetics

34. Which drug could be used for seizures and wound healing?
   a. phenytoin (Dilantin)
   b. chlorhexadine gluconate (Hibiclens)
   c. crotamiton (Eurax)
   d. carbamide peroxide (Gly-Oxide Oral)

35. What is the most commonly occurring eye disease?
   a. conjunctivitis (dry eye)
   b. cataracts
   c. glaucoma
   d. CMV retinitis

36. Which of the following is a precancerous condition?
   a. basal cell carcinoma
   b. keratoacanthoma
   c. melanoma
   d. actinic keratosis

37. Local freezing can be used to treat
   a. dandruff.
   b. warts.
   c. unwanted facial hair.
   d. ringworm.
   e. actinic keratosis.

38. Which of the following bacterial skin infections is characterized by blisters and encrustations?
   a. erysipelas
   b. impetigo
   c. folliculitis
   d. furuncle

39. What term describes a small circular ring of DNA that can be used to transfer a gene to a host cell?
   a. ligase
   b. monoclonal antibody
   c. promotor
   d. plasmid

40. Centruroides (Scorpion) immune F is approved for
    a. scorpion stings
    b. mosquito bites
    c. spider bites
    d. tick bites

41. Which statement is not true regarding probiotics?
    a. they stimulate the growth of beneficial bacteria in the body
    b. they are a good laxative
    c. they are "good" bacteria
    d. some yogurt is a probiotic

42. What is the advantage of recombinant DNA technology?
    a. It can produce pure human protein in large quantities.
    b. It can produce pure human protein without the risk of viral contamination.
    c. It can produce pure human protein far less expensively than traditional technology.
    d. a and b
    e. a, b, and c

43. What vitamin found in dairy products, liver, and fish oils is also known as retinol?
    a. vitamin A
    b. vitamin D_2
    c. vitamin E
    d. vitamin K

44. Which of the following drugs may cause tinnitus (ringing in the ear), nausea, and vomiting in children with doses greater than 150 mg/kg?
    a. tricyclic antidepressants
    b. aspirin
    c. morphine
    d. acetaminophen (Tylenol)

45. What reversal agent may be used to treat narcotic respiratory depression?
    a. edetate calcium disodium (Calcium Disodium Versenate)
    b. phentolamine (Regitine)
    c. naloxone (Narcan)
    d. glucagon (GlucaGen)

46. Which of the following statements is true about vitamins?
    a. They are organic substances required for metabolic functions.
    b. They cannot be converted to coenzymes in the body.
    c. The body can synthesize sufficient amounts of some vitamins.
    d. They are proteins that assist in performing metabolic functions.

47. A bioterrorism attack may include
    a. emerging infectious diseases
    b. biologic agents
    c. interactions
    d. a and b
    e. all of the above

48. Malnutrition can lead to all of the below, except
    a. poor wound healing
    b. infections
    c. hair growth
    d. organ system failure
    e. decrease in body stores of calories to protein

49. Which of the following are issues involving alternative supplements?
    a. mistaken identity
    b. forgoing professional treatment
    c. interactions
    d. a and b
    e. a, b, and c

50. What is the pharmacy technician's responsibility when a Blue Alert cart is returned to the pharmacy?
    a. Restock drugs.
    b. Remove and replace expired drugs.
    c. Remove and replace drugs that will expire in the next month.
    d. a and b
    e. a, b, and c

Final Exam

Multiple Choice

Identify the choice that best completes the statement or answers the question.

1. The PTCB is
   a. an organization of educators that focuses on pharmacy technnician training curriculums and networking
   b. an organization that maintains a national certification program for technicians
   c. composed of pharmacy technicians and provides leadership
   d. an agency of the federal government responsible for ensuring safety of drugs
   e. a branch of the federal government responsible for regulating the sale of drugs

2. What is the source of pepsin?
   a. plants
   b. animal products
   c. minerals
   d. synthetic materials
   e. bioengineering

3. Alternative medicines, including herbs, supplements, and homeopathic remedies
   a. have been tested and approved by the FDA.
   b. should not be taken by patients.
   c. are bioequivalent from manufacturer to manufacturer.
   d. can interact adversely with prescription drugs.
   e. All of the above

4. What determines the order in which the FDA processes New Drug Applications?
   a. availability of review teams
   b. "first-come, first-served" basis
   c. results of clinical trials
   d. seriousness of the targeted disease

5. Professionals and consumers can report serious adverse drug reactions to
   a. MedWatch.
   b. the DEA.
   c. the USP-NF.
   d. the PTCB.
   e. the NABP.

6. What is the rate-limiting factor for drug distribution?
   a. acidity of drug
   b. patient disease state
   c. blood-brain barrier
   d. blood flow
   e. drug chemistry

7. What does bioavailability reflect?
   a. the fraction of an administered dose that is available to the target tissue
   b. the amount of drug, given intravenously, that enters the bloodstream
   c. the amount of drug absorbed by the liver
   d. the amount of drug absorbed by the kidneys
   e. the maximal effect produced by a drug

8. If a drug has a half-life of 6 hours and a starting blood concentration of 100 mg/kg, how long will it take until the concentration of the drug in blood is 25 mg/kg?
   a. 3 hours
   b. 6 hours
   c. 12 hours
   d. 24 hours

9. Which statement is *not* true about receptors?
   a. Receptors are protein molecules.
   b. Receptors are located in extra-cellular fluid.
   c. There are different types of receptors throughout the body.
   d. Receptors and chemical messengers must have complementary structures to bind.
   e. Receptors play a role in blood clotting and smooth muscle contraction.

10. What statement is *true* about lipids?
    a. They are protein molecules.
    b. They generally attract water.
    c. They generally repel water.
    d. They are not part of the cell membrane.

11. What is the advantage of metabolizing drugs to more water-soluble forms?
    a. Water-soluble forms can more readily be excreted by the kidneys.
    b. Water-soluble forms can more readily be excreted by the liver.
    c. Water-soluble forms can increase the rate of gastric emptying.
    d. Water-soluble forms can pass through the blood-brain barrier.
    e. Water-soluble forms can decrease the amount of drug lost to protein binding.

12. Loading doses may be accomplished by
    a. a single large dose.
    b. a series of doses.
    c. doubling the maintenance dose.
    d. decreasing the maintenance dose.
    e. a, b, and c

13. The label "Do not take with antacids" is placed on a prescription container to warn patients of a potential
    a. drug interaction.
    b. allergic response.
    c. adverse side effect.
    d. a and b
    e. a, b, and c

14. What route is often used if a patient is experiencing nausea and vomiting and parenteral administration is not desired (provided this dosage form is available)?
    a. intrathecal
    b. rectal
    c. sublingual
    d. po
    e. vaginal

15. Which abbreviation should a prescriber use to indicate that a patient is to take the medication before meals?
    a. qd
    b. qh
    c. ud
    d. tid
    e. ac

16. Why is parenteral administration necessary for some drugs?
    a. They must be swallowed to become effective.
    b. They must pass through the liver.
    c. They are excreted by the kidneys.
    d. They are inactivated by digestive juices.

17. When dispensing a new medication, the pharmacy technician should ask the patient,
    a. "Are your address and phone number current?"
    b. "Do you have health insurance?"
    c. "When is your birthday?"
    d. "Do you have any allergies?"
    e. All of the above

18. The removal of a drug or its metabolites from the body is
    a. absorption
    b. distribution
    c. metabolism
    d. induction
    e. elimination

19. What is the biggest challenge in developing a new antibiotic?
    a. keeping the cost as low as possible
    b. finding a way to make the drug water soluble
    c. killing the bacteria without harming the patient
    d. assuring distribution to all tissues in the body including heart, brain, and muscle
    e. making sure it is bactericidal

20. The ceiling effect occurs when
    a. a disease, symptom, or condition benefits from the drug
    b. when a drug increases the concentration of enzymes that affect the pharmacological response
    c. no clinical response occurs with increased dosage
    d. an unusual or unexpected response occurs

21. Which of the following drugs is classified as a macrolide?
a. penicillin V
b. tetracycline
c. erythromycin
d. ciprofloxacin
e. telithromycin

22. __________ works by conversion of metabolic processes within the body.
a. prodrug
b. penicillin
c. aminoglycoside
d. superinfection
e. sepsis

23. What color would *Escherichia coli* turn during Gram staining?
a. red
b. green
c. yellow
d. orange
e. purple

24. What auxiliary label on antibiotic prescriptions might help to reduce antimicrobial resistance?
a. Take with fluids.
b. Avoid sun exposure.
c. Take all of this medication.
d. Do not drink alcoholic beverages while taking this medication.
e. Take on an empty stomach.

25. Sulfonamides are commonly used to treat
a. venereal diseases.
b. abscesses.
c. heart valve infections.
d. urinary tract infections.
e. a and d

26. Which class of drugs could result in an adverse drug interaction if taken with daptomycin (Cubicin), a cyclic lipopeptide?
a. calcium channel blockers
b. antihistamines
c. statins
d. corticosteroids
e. bronchodilators

27. What is a common target of fungal infections?
a. brain
b. heart
c. lungs
d. ears
e. nails

28. HAART is
a. capsid
b. regimen for HIV that has reduced morbidity and mortality
c. naked virus
d. interferon

29. Which of the following statements is true?
a. Viruses are easily avoided.
b. A virus replicates within a living host cell.
c. A virion will contain both RNA and DNA.
d. A virus without a capsid is called a naked virus.
e. b and d

30. What is the last stage of a viral infection?
a. The virus escapes into the cytoplasm.
b. The virus takes over the host cell nuclear activity.
c. The virus attaches to a cell receptor.
d. The virus uncoats and sheds its covering.
e. The cell membrane closes around the virus.

31. Prior to administering a flu shot, it is important to confirm that the patient is *not* allergic to
a. horse serum.
b. needles.
c. peanuts.
d. dust mites.
e. eggs.

32. Following injection with a local anesthetic, what sensation is affected first?
a. temperature perception
b. pain perception
c. skeletal muscle tone
d. consciousness

33. Which of the following narcotics is a controlled substance?
   a. morphine
   b. codeine
   c. oxycodone (OxyContin)
   d. meperidine (Demerol)
   e. All of the above

34. A pain that occurs when no pain should be felt is
   a. somatic.
   b. chronic malignant.
   c. acute.
   d. sympathetically mediated.

35. Which of the following drugs is classified as a tricyclic antidepressant and has significant anticholinergic side effects?
   a. lithium (Eskalith)
   b. imipramine (Tofranil)
   c. fluoxetine (Prozac)
   d. venlafaxine (Effexor)

36. Which monoamine oxidase inhibitor is used to treat Parkinson patients rather than depressed patients?
   a. phenelzine (Nardil)
   b. tranylcypromine (Parnate)
   c. selegiline (Eldepryl)
   d. buproprion (Wellbutrin)

37. What is a good indication that the patient is taking a therapeutic dose of lithium?
   a. washing hands over and over
   b. anxiety attacks
   c. strange sexual behaviors
   d. slight tremor of hands

38. Which benzodiazepine is *not* approved for sleep disorders?
   a. flurazepam (Dalmane)
   b. triazolam (Halcion)
   c. zolpidem (Ambien)
   d. diazepam (Valium)

39. Which anticonvulsant is the drug of choice for absence seizures?
   a. lorazepam (Ativan)
   b. valproic acid (Depakene)
   c. lamotrigine (Lamictal)
   d. ethosuximide (Zarontin)

40. A generalized seizure
   a. is the most common type of seizure.
   b. occurs in two distinct types.
   c. involves both hemispheres of the brain simultaneously.
   d. may progress to a partial seizure.

41. Which anti-Parkinson agent is associated with the on-off phenomenon?
   a. levodopa (Dopar)
   b. bromocriptine (Parlodel)
   c. pergolide (Permax)
   d. tolcapone (Tasmar)
   e. ropinirole (ReQuip)

42. Which drug is approved to treat Huntington's Chorea?
   a. Lyrica (pregabalin)
   b. Topamax (topiramate)
   c. Symmetrel (amantadine)
   d. Xenazine (tetrabenazine)

43. Why might a prescribing physician prefer donepezil (Aricept) over tacrine (Cognex) for Alzheimer disease?
   a. Donepezil is given once a day.
   b. Donepezil does not result in nausea, vomiting, and diarrhea.
   c. Donepezil improves memory and alertness.
   d. a and b
   e. a, b, and c

44. Which of the following is a potentially life-threatening condition in which the patient has difficulty breathing, has blue lips and nail beds, may lose consciousness, and does not respond to normal management?
   a. status emphysema
   b. chronic bronchitis
   c. status asthmaticus
   d. acute bronchitis

45. What is the *least*-sedating OTC antihistamine and the only one approved by the FDA for cold symptoms?
   a. fexofenadine (Allegra)
   b. loratadine (Claritin)
   c. desloratadine (Clarinex)
   d. clemastine (Tavist Allergy)
   e. azelastine (Astelin, Optivar)

46. Emphysema is a pulmonary disease that
   a. is reversible.
   b. obstructs air flow on inspiration.
   c. destroys the tiny air sacs of the lungs.
   d. a and b
   e. a, b, and c

47. Histoplasmosis is transmitted by
   a. having hand contact with an infected person.
   b. inhaling bacteria-laden drops.
   c. breathing in fungus-bearing dust.
   d. inheriting the gene for the disease from one's parents.

48. Why do pharmacies in many areas of the country currently limit the sale of pseudoephedrine (Sudafed)?
   a. Pseudoephedrine is a different name for ephedrine.
   b. Pseudoephedrine is in short supply.
   c. Pseudoephedrine has abuse potential.
   d. Pseudoephedrine has many adverse side effects.
   e. Pseudoephedrine has questionable efficacy.

49. Which of the following gives correct instructions for using the nicotine patch?
   a. Apply a new patch weekly.
   b. Apply to a nonhairy, clean, dry site.
   c. Use the same application site.
   d. Apply to the lower body or outer leg.

50. Which histamine$_2$ receptor blocker affects the cytochrome P-450 system and may interact with many other drugs?
   a. ranitidine (Zantac)
   b. famotidine (Pepcid)
   c. lansoprazole (Prevacid)
   d. cimetidine (Tagamet)

51. What group of drugs is the mainstay of treatment for *H. pylori*?
   a. antacids
   b. H_2 blockers
   c. antibiotics
   d. a and c
   e. All of the above

52. What GI disorder is characterized by inflammation of the large bowel with the patient experiencing diarrhea containing blood, mucus, and pus?
   a. ulcerative colitis
   b. gastritis
   c. gastroesophageal reflux disease (GERD)
   d. malabsorption syndrome

53. By what criterion is dietary fiber characterized?
   a. fermentability
   b. water-holding capacity
   c. stool-bulking capacity
   d. solubility
   e. All of the above

54. Which of the following drugs is used for chemotherapy-induced emesis and frequently causes headaches in patients treated with it?
   a. ondansetron (Zofran)
   b. sibutramine (Meridia)
   c. primaquine
   d. prochlorperazine (Compazine)

55. What is praziquantel (Biltricide) used to treat?
   a. intestinal parasites (tapeworms)
   b. amebiasis caused by *Entamoeba histolytica*
   c. malaria
   d. hepatitis

56. Which antihistamine is not an H-2 blocker?
   a. Tagamet (cimetidiine)
   b. Benadryl (diphenhydramine)
   c. Axid (nizatidine)
   d. Zantac (ranitidine)
   e. Pepcid (famotidine)

57. Patients in the intensive care unit are frequently given H_2 blockers to prevent the development of
   a. GERD.
   b. ulcerative colitis.
   c. stress ulcers.
   d. drug-induced ulcers.

58. An infection of malaria can be acquired by way of
    a. mosquitoes.
    b. sharing needles.
    c. a blood transfusion from an infected donor.
    d. a and b
    e. a, b, and c

59. What is a goal of renal therapy?
    a. reestablishing an appropriate intravascular volume
    b. restricting fluids in volume-overload patients
    c. treating underlying fluid, electrolyte, or pH problems
    d. All of the above

60. Which group has the highest incidence of urinary tract infections?
    a. older men
    b. sexually active women
    c. bed-wetting children
    d. athletes
    e. postmenopausal women

61. Which of the following is a urinary tract infection of the upper tract?
    a. cystitis
    b. urethritis
    c. prostatitis
    d. pyelonephritis

62. What warning label should accompany alfuzosin (Uroxatral)?
    a. Take 1 hour before eating.
    b. Take with fluids.
    c. Take on an empty stomach.
    d. Do not chew, split, or crush.
    e. Take with food.

63. What does the systolic blood pressure reading represent?
    a. pressure during the filling of the heart
    b. pressure after the heart has emptied
    c. total peripheral resistance
    d. cardiac output

64. Which of the antiplatelet drugs listed below is a monoclonal antibody?
    a. abciximab (ReoPro)
    b. eptifibatide (Integrilin)
    c. tirofiban (Aggrastat)
    d. clopidogrel (Plavix)

65. If circulation of oxygen to the brain is stopped, how long will it take for the brain to use up its supply of oxygen?
    a. 5 seconds
    b. 10 seconds
    c. 15 seconds
    d. 20 seconds

66. Which of the following drugs reduces cholesterol levels by inhibiting HMG-CoA reductase, the enzyme that catalyzes the rate-limiting step in the synthesis of cholesterol?
    a. gemfibrozil (Lopid)
    b. simvastatin (Zocor)
    c. niacin (Simcor)
    d. ezetimibe (Zetia)

67. Which disease is a risk factor for heart problems?
    a. cancer
    b. arthritis
    c. diabetes
    d. epilepsy
    e. asthma

68. Why do many patients with congestive heart failure resist taking ACE inhibitors?
    a. ACE inhibitors produce a persistent and annoying cough.
    b. ACE inhibitors must be dosed three times daily.
    c. ACE inhibitors present a risk of hypokalemia.
    d. ACE inhibitors are among the most costly drugs for treating cardiovascular disease.

69. Which heart problem is the leading cause of death in industrialized nations?
    a. arrhythmia
    b. congestive heart failure
    c. myocardial infarction
    d. angina
    e. hypertension

70. Which type of stroke involves primary rupture of a blood vessel?
    a. ischemic
    b. transient
    c. hemorrhagic
    d. reversible

71. The lethal dose of aspirin for an adult is usually more than
   a. 650 mg.
   b. 1 g.
   c. 3.5 g.
   d. 10 g.

72. What prostaglandin molecule, which facilitates platelet aggregation, is inhibited by low dose (81–325 mg) aspirin?
   a. thromboxane A2
   b. prostacyclin
   c. PGE2
   d. cyclooxygenase

73. Which of the following drugs is *least* likely to produce GI irritation at analgesic doses?
   a. naproxen (Aleve, Anaprox, Naprosyn)
   b. sulindac (Clinoril)
   c. aspirin
   d. celecoxib (Celebrex)

74. What auxiliary sticker should be on every NSAID?
   a. stay out of the sun
   b. take with a full glass of water
   c. take with food
   d. store in the refrigerator
   e. do not drink alcohol

75. Which of the following statements about NSAIDs is *not* true?
   a. NSAIDs act centrally, rather than peripherally.
   b. NSAIDs take longer to reduce fever than other products.
   c. NSAIDs inhibit PG synthesis in inflamed tissues.
   d. NSAIDs often lead to some type of gastropathy.

76. Which NSAID has an oral liquid form and is suitable for children?
   a. naproxen (Aleve)
   b. ibuprofen (Advil, Motrin)
   c. mefenamic acid (Ponstel)
   d. etodolac (Lodine)
   e. buffered aspirin (Bufferin)

77. What NSAID is the most used for gouty arthritis?
   a. sulfinpyrazone (Anturane)
   b. indomethacin (Indocin)
   c. allopurinol (Zyloprim)
   d. colchicine

78. Which of the following antibiotics is often the drug of choice for treating syphilis?
   a. penicillin G benzathine (Bicillin L-A)
   b. ketoconazole (Nizoral)
   c. valacyclovir (Valtrex)
   d. azithromycin (Zithromax)
   e. tertacycline (Sumycin)

79. Which synthetic insulin is the longest acting?
   a. lispro (Humalog)
   b. aspart (Novolog)
   c. NPH (Humulin N)
   d. glargine (Lantus)

80. Combined estrogen-progestin oral contraceptives prevent conception by
   a. interfering with the production of the hormones that regulate the menstrual cycle.
   b. altering the cervical mucus to form a physical barrier that prevents the penetration of sperm.
   c. changing the composition of the endometrium to make it unsuitable for implantation.
   d. a and b
   e. a, b, and c

81. What is needed for calcium to absorbed into bone tissue?
   a. vitamin A
   b. vitamin B
   c. vitamin C
   d. vitamin D
   e. vitamin E

82. Which of the following is a type of sweat gland?
   a. eccrine
   b. endocrine
   c. epocrine
   d. sebaceous

83. What term is used to describe the excessive response of the skin to sun in the presence of a sensitizing agent?
   a. photoreactivity
   b. photosensitivity
   c. photoconductivity
   d. acne

84. Which ear medication is specifically to alleviate pain?
   a. ciprofloxin
   b. hydrocortisone
   c. antipytine-benzocaine
   d. carbamide peroxide

85. What term defines chemicals that free objects of pathogenic organisms or render the organisms inert?
   a. disinfectant
   b. germicide
   c. preservative
   d. sanitizer

86. What is a major characteristic of eczema, or dermatitis?
   a. melanoma
   b. sebum
   c. pruritus
   d. urticaria

87. Which of the following skin disorders is a fungal infection?
   a. dandruff
   b. cellulitis
   c. psoriasis
   d. candidiasis
   e. dermatitis

88. Which class of drugs is typically used to treat poison ivy?
   a. antibiotics
   b. corticosteroids
   c. antihistamines
   d. b and c

89. Which of the following might a parent use to treat a child's scraped knee?
   a. benzocaine (Hurricaine)
   b. clove oil (Eugenol)
   c. benzalkonium chloride (Zephiran)
   d. alcohol
   e. povidone-iodine (Betadine)

90. The pharmacy technician should inform the pharmacist if
   a. the physician prescribes eardrops for an eye infection.
   b. the physician prescribes an otic antibiotic but not an accompanying pain reliever.
   c. the physician prescribes an otic solution for a patient with a tube in the ear.
   d. a and b
   e. a, b, and c

91. A cytoprotective agent is used to
   a. reduce the side effects and toxicity of chemotherapy agents
   b. leads to DNA damage when cells replicate
   c. direct attacks against specific objectives
   d. inhibit the formation of spindle fibers

92. Timing is critical when administering a rescue agent because it
   a. reduces side effects
   b. prevents the destruction of healthy cells
   c. completes the course of the medication
   d. prevents oral complications

93. What drug is used to treat Hodgkin disease?
   a. imatinib (Gleevec)
   b. gefitnib (Iressa)
   c. pemetrexad (Alimta)
   d. procarbazine (Matulane)

94. What is the part of DNA where protein production starts?
   a. promoter sequence
   b. terminator sequence
   c. RNA polymerase
   d. nucleotide bases

95. Which of the following drugs may cause tinnitus (ringing in the ear), nausea, and vomiting in children with doses greater than 150 mg/kg?
   a. tricyclic antidepressants
   b. aspirin
   c. morphine
   d. acetaminophen (Tylenol)

96. Before dispensing medications to treat or prevent the effects of a bioterrorism outbreak, a pharmacy technician should
   a. point out possible drug interactions.
   b. answer questions about the medication.
   c. explain how to take the medication.
   d. identify patient allergies.

97. Which of the following statements is true about vitamins?
   a. They are organic substances required for metabolic functions.
   b. They cannot be converted to coenzymes in the body.
   c. The body can synthesize sufficient amounts of some vitamins.
   d. They are proteins that assist in performing metabolic functions.

98. Alcoholics are often deficient in
   a. vitamin B_1.
   b. vitamin B_9.
   c. vitamin B_{12}.
   d. a and b
   e. a, b, and c

99. Which herb might benefit patients with diabetes?
   a. chromium picolinate
   b. glucosamine sulfate
   c. ginseng
   d. feverfew
   e. valerian

100. Which drug do some physicians prescribe to try to preserve the skin around the bite of a brown recluse spider?
   a. sodium nitrate
   b. atropine
   c. physostigmine
   d. dapsone

Answers

Chapter 1 Quiz

1. ANS: C p. 4
2. ANS: D pp. 4, 20
3. ANS: C p. 6
4. ANS: B p. 6
5. ANS: B p. 11
6. ANS: A p. 12
7. ANS: D p. 14
8. ANS: B p. 14
9. ANS: A p. 15
10. ANS: D p. 17
11. ANS: B p. 18
12. ANS: A p. 19
13. ANS: B p. 10
14. ANS: B p. 5
15. ANS: B p. 7
16. ANS: E p. 8
17. ANS: B p. 11
18. ANS: A p. 15
19. ANS: D p. 16
20. ANS: E p. 18

Chapter 2 Quiz

1. ANS: D p. 27
2. ANS: D pp. 27–29
3. ANS: B p. 28
4. ANS: D pp. 29, 36
5. ANS: B pp. 30, 35
6. ANS: C pp. 31–32, 35
7. ANS: C pp. 31–32
8. ANS: B pp. 32, 35
9. ANS: B pp. 26, 36
10. ANS: C p. 26
11. ANS: D p. 27
12. ANS: A p. 27
13. ANS: C p. 28
14. ANS: C pp. 29, 35
15. ANS: C p. 30
16. ANS: D pp. 31, 36
17. ANS: B p. 31
18. ANS: C p. 33
19. ANS: A p. 34
20. ANS: C p. 34

Chapter 3 Quiz

1. ANS: A p. 41
2. ANS: D p. 42
3. ANS: C p. 46
4. ANS: C p. 48
5. ANS: B p. 49
6. ANS: E pp. 49–50
7. ANS: B pp. 53, 63
8. ANS: A p. 57
9. ANS: C p. 42
10. ANS: A p. 46
11. ANS: C p. 46
12. ANS: C pp. 48, 63
13. ANS: A p. 50
14. ANS: C p. 50
15. ANS: D p. 53
16. ANS: A pp. 53, 63
17. ANS: B pp. 53, 63
18. ANS: A p. 54
19. ANS: A p. 60
20. ANS: B p. 60

Chapter 4 Quiz

Answer Section

Multiple Choice

1. ANS: A p. 75
2. ANS: C pp. 73, 93
3. ANS: B pp. 73, 93
4. ANS: B p. 74
5. ANS: C p. 74
6. ANS: C p. 87
7. ANS: B p. 88
8. ANS: D p. 90
9. ANS: D p. 98
10. ANS: C p. 83
11. ANS: A p. 85
12. ANS: D p. 91
13. ANS: C p. 74
14. ANS: B p. 76
15. ANS: D pp. 77, 95
16. ANS: A pp. 83, 96
17. ANS: C p. 93
18. ANS: A p. 88
19. ANS: B p. 89
20. ANS: D p. 92

Chapter 5 Quiz

Answer Section

Multiple Choice

1. ANS: B p. 103
2. ANS: C p. 104
3. ANS: B p. 106
4. ANS: A p. 106
5. ANS: C p. 107
6. ANS: D pp. 109–110
7. ANS: D p. 112
8. ANS: D p. 112
9. ANS: A pp. 112–113
10. ANS: E p. 128
11. ANS: A p. 119
12. ANS: B p. 106
13. ANS: B p. 105
14. ANS: B p. 113
15. ANS: B p. 108
16. ANS: E p. 109
17. ANS: A p. 110
18. ANS: C p. 113
19. ANS: D p. 117
20. ANS: D p. 125

Chapter 6 Quiz

Answer Section

Multiple Choice

1. ANS: E p. 134
2. ANS: D p. 134
3. ANS: C p. 138

4.	ANS:	A	p. 167
5.	ANS:	D	p. 143
6.	ANS:	B	p. 148
7.	ANS:	D	p. 160
8.	ANS:	D	p. 160
9.	ANS:	B	p. 134
10.	ANS:	C	p. 135
11.	ANS:	D	p. 136
12.	ANS:	A	p. 139
13.	ANS:	B	pp. 139–140
14.	ANS:	D	p. 147
15.	ANS:	C	p. 149
16.	ANS:	C	p. 151
17.	ANS:	C	p. 159
18.	ANS:	E	pp. 159, 166
19.	ANS:	E	p. 161
20.	ANS:	A	p. 163

Chapter 7 Quiz

Answer Section

Multiple Choice

1.	ANS:	A	p. 174
2.	ANS:	A	p. 177
3.	ANS:	B	p. 180
4.	ANS:	D	p. 182
5.	ANS:	D	p. 182
6.	ANS:	B	p. 185
7.	ANS:	D	p. 186
8.	ANS:	C	p. 191
9.	ANS:	D	p. 193
10.	ANS:	C	p. 196
11.	ANS:	B	p. 174
12.	ANS:	C	p. 178
13.	ANS:	C	p. 179
14.	ANS:	E	p. 182
15.	ANS:	C	p. 183
16.	ANS:	B	p. 182
17.	ANS:	C	p. 183
18.	ANS:	C	p. 185
19.	ANS:	A	p. 191
20.	ANS:	D	p. 195

Chapter 8 Quiz

Answer Section

Multiple Choice

1.	ANS:	D	p. 208
2.	ANS:	D	p. 209
3.	ANS:	E	p. 212
4.	ANS:	E	p. 211
5.	ANS:	C	p. 212
6.	ANS:	B	p. 213
7.	ANS:	E	p. 217
8.	ANS:	E	p. 223
9.	ANS:	C	p. 225
10.	ANS:	C	pp. 208, 229
11.	ANS:	C	p. 209
12.	ANS:	D	p. 210
13.	ANS:	A	p. 218
14.	ANS:	C	pp. 220–221
15.	ANS:	B	p. 228
16.	ANS:	D	pp. 227, 232
17.	ANS:	B	p. 225
18.	ANS:	E	p. 226
19.	ANS:	A	p. 226
20.	ANS:	C	p. 226

Chapter 9 Quiz

Answer Section

Multiple Choice

1.	ANS:	B	p. 237
2.	ANS:	C	p. 238
3.	ANS:	B	p. 240
4.	ANS:	D	p. 243
5.	ANS:	D	p. 246
6.	ANS:	A	p. 259
7.	ANS:	E	p. 267
8.	ANS:	B	p. 245
9.	ANS:	B	p. 247
10.	ANS:	C	p. 248
11.	ANS:	A	p. 251
12.	ANS:	B	p. 254
13.	ANS:	B	p. 254
14.	ANS:	C	p. 255
15.	ANS:	D	p. 257
16.	ANS:	D	p. 263
17.	ANS:	A	p. 264
18.	ANS:	B	p. 266
19.	ANS:	A	p. 268
20.	ANS:	B	p. 269

Chapter 10 Quiz

Answer Section

Multiple Choice

1.	ANS:	E	p. 284
2.	ANS:	E	p. 289
3.	ANS:	D	p. 290
4.	ANS:	B	p. 291
5.	ANS:	A	p. 294
6.	ANS:	B	p. 295
7.	ANS:	D	p. 295
8.	ANS:	D	p. 300
9.	ANS:	D	p. 300
10.	ANS:	A	p. 305
11.	ANS:	A	pp. 310, 321
12.	ANS:	A	p. 312
13.	ANS:	E	p. 283
14.	ANS:	B	p. 284
15.	ANS:	A	p. 294
16.	ANS:	D	pp. 295–296
17.	ANS:	A	p. 308
18.	ANS:	B	pp. 309–310, 316
19.	ANS:	C	p. 316
20.	ANS:	B	p. 310

Chapter 11 Quiz

Answer Section

Multiple Choice

1.	ANS:	C	p. 326
2.	ANS:	E	p. 326
3.	ANS:	D	p. 326
4.	ANS:	D	p. 329
5.	ANS:	B	p. 329
6.	ANS:	C	pp. 333–334
7.	ANS:	D	p. 335
8.	ANS:	E	pp. 335–336
9.	ANS:	A	p. 336
10.	ANS:	B	p. 338

11.	ANS:	B	p. 329
12.	ANS:	B	p. 326
13.	ANS:	B	p. 327
14.	ANS:	B	p. 329
15.	ANS:	D	p. 332
16.	ANS:	B	p. 334
17.	ANS:	D	p. 334
18.	ANS:	A	p. 335
19.	ANS:	C	p. 336
20.	ANS:	C	p. 341

Chapter 12 Quiz

Answer Section

Multiple Choice

1.	ANS:	B	p. 352
2.	ANS:	D	p. 353
3.	ANS:	D	p. 356
4.	ANS:	D	p. 356
5.	ANS:	D	p. 363
6.	ANS:	C	p. 365
7.	ANS:	A	p. 374
8.	ANS:	A	pp. 372–374
9.	ANS:	C	p. 377
10.	ANS:	D	p. 380
11.	ANS:	B	p. 384
12.	ANS:	A	p. 384
13.	ANS:	B	p. 386
14.	ANS:	C	p. 392
15.	ANS:	B	pp. 361, 396
16.	ANS:	B	p. 365
17.	ANS:	A	p. 371
18.	ANS:	D	p. 379
19.	ANS:	D	p. 389
20.	ANS:	C	p. 392

Chapter 13 Quiz

Answer Section

Multiple Choice

1.	ANS:	D	p. 411
2.	ANS:	B	p. 412
3.	ANS:	B	p. 414
4.	ANS:	A	p. 414
5.	ANS:	C	p. 415
6.	ANS:	A	p. 415
7.	ANS:	A	p. 415
8.	ANS:	C	p. 419
9.	ANS:	D	p. 422
10.	ANS:	C	p. 407
11.	ANS:	B	p. 408
12.	ANS:	A	p. 411
13.	ANS:	D	p. 411
14.	ANS:	C	p. 412
15.	ANS:	D	p. 413
16.	ANS:	A	pp. 417, 429
17.	ANS:	B	p. 417
18.	ANS:	C	p. 419
19.	ANS:	B	p. 421
20.	ANS:	A	p. 426

Chapter 14 Quiz

Answer Section

Multiple Choice

1.	ANS:	D	p. 440
2.	ANS:	E	pp. 443–444
3.	ANS:	B	p. 454
4.	ANS:	E	p. 455
5.	ANS:	A	pp. 112, 462
6.	ANS:	A	p. 467
7.	ANS:	D	p. 472
8.	ANS:	E	p. 442
9.	ANS:	A	p. 443
10.	ANS:	E	p. 443
11.	ANS:	C	p. 448
12.	ANS:	E	p. 450
13.	ANS:	A	p. 457
14.	ANS:	D	p. 458
15.	ANS:	D	p. 466
16.	ANS:	C	p. 446
17.	ANS:	C	p. 468
18.	ANS:	D	p. 469
19.	ANS:	B	p. 471
20.	ANS:	A	p. 480

Chapter 15 Quiz

Answer Section

Multiple Choice

1.	ANS:	C	p. 493
2.	ANS:	B	p. 495
3.	ANS:	D	p. 504
4.	ANS:	D	p. 500
5.	ANS:	B	p. 506
6.	ANS:	B	p. 514
7.	ANS:	A	p. 518
8.	ANS:	B	p. 521
9.	ANS:	D	p. 521
10.	ANS:	A	p. 522
11.	ANS:	D	p. 526
12.	ANS:	A	p. 524
13.	ANS:	B	p. 495
14.	ANS:	B	p. 506
15.	ANS:	B	p. 506
16.	ANS:	D	p. 502
17.	ANS:	B	p. 511
18.	ANS:	A	p. 524
19.	ANS:	D	p. 510
20.	ANS:	E	p. 525

Chapter 16 Quiz

Answer Section

Multiple Choice

1.	ANS:	A	p. 544
2.	ANS:	C	p. 545
3.	ANS:	A	p. 545
4.	ANS:	C	p. 546
5.	ANS:	B	p. 548
6.	ANS:	C	p. 549
7.	ANS:	E	p. 550
8.	ANS:	B	p. 551
9.	ANS:	D	p. 565
10.	ANS:	C	p. 568
11.	ANS:	D	p. 541
12.	ANS:	A	p. 541
13.	ANS:	A	p. 543
14.	ANS:	C	p. 574
15.	ANS:	C	p. 547
16.	ANS:	C	p. 553

17.	ANS:	B	p. 513
18.	ANS:	D	p. 555
19.	ANS:	E	p. 556
20.	ANS:	D	p. 566

Chapter 17 Quiz

Answer Section

Multiple Choice

1.	ANS:	B	p. 580
2.	ANS:	A	p. 581
3.	ANS:	D	p. 583
4.	ANS:	A	p. 586
5.	ANS:	A	p. 587
6.	ANS:	B	p. 589
7.	ANS:	B	p. 597
8.	ANS:	B	p. 600
9.	ANS:	C	p. 600
10.	ANS:	E	p. 606
11.	ANS:	E	p. 580
12.	ANS:	E	p. 582
13.	ANS:	E	p. 584
14.	ANS:	E	p. 589
15.	ANS:	B	p. 591
16.	ANS:	C	p. 591
17.	ANS:	C	p. 597
18.	ANS:	D	p. 598
19.	ANS:	B	p. 601
20.	ANS:	E	p. 607

Unit 1 Test

Answer Section

Multiple Choice

1.	ANS:	B	p. 6
2.	ANS:	B	p. 11
3.	ANS:	A	p. 14
4.	ANS:	A	p. 15
5.	ANS:	B	p. 18
6.	ANS:	A	p. 19
7.	ANS:	D	p. 5
8.	ANS:	B	p. 5
9.	ANS:	C	p. 7
10.	ANS:	E	p. 8
11.	ANS:	C	p. 12
12.	ANS:	A	p. 15
13.	ANS:	D	p. 16
14.	ANS:	E	p. 18
15.	ANS:	C	p. 19
16.	ANS:	D	pp. 26, 35
17.	ANS:	B	pp. 27, 36
18.	ANS:	C	p. 29
19.	ANS:	A	p. 31
20.	ANS:	B	p. 154
21.	ANS:	C	p. 34
22.	ANS:	C	p. 34
23.	ANS:	D	p. 47
24.	ANS:	C	p. 29
25.	ANS:	E	p. 30
26.	ANS:	C	p. 47
27.	ANS:	D	pp. 31, 36
28.	ANS:	B	pp. 33, 36
29.	ANS:	C	p. 46
30.	ANS:	E	p. 50
31.	ANS:	E	p. 43
32.	ANS:	D	p. 46
33.	ANS:	A	p. 46
34.	ANS:	E	p. 60
35.	ANS:	C	p. 49
36.	ANS:	A	p. 55
37.	ANS:	B	p. 57
38.	ANS:	D	p. 57
39.	ANS:	A	p. 57
40.	ANS:	B	p. 60

Unit 2 Test

Answer Section

Multiple Choice

1.	ANS:	E	p. 73
2.	ANS:	C	pp. 73, 93
3.	ANS:	C	pp. 73, 75
4.	ANS:	B	p. 88
5.	ANS:	D	p. 75
6.	ANS:	D	p. 76
7.	ANS:	A	p. 79
8.	ANS:	D	p. 105
9.	ANS:	D	p. 105
10.	ANS:	C	p. 107
11.	ANS:	B	p. 106
12.	ANS:	D	p. 109
13.	ANS:	D	p. 112
14.	ANS:	D	p. 112
15.	ANS:	E	p. 128
16.	ANS:	E	p. 114
17.	ANS:	A	p. 128
18.	ANS:	C	p. 134
19.	ANS:	D	p. 158
20.	ANS:	B	p. 139
21.	ANS:	A	p. 153
22.	ANS:	D	p. 142
23.	ANS:	D	p. 145
24.	ANS:	C	p. 151
25.	ANS:	D	p. 162
26.	ANS:	A	p. 163
27.	ANS:	D	p. 183
28.	ANS:	C	p. 193
29.	ANS:	C	p. 179
30.	ANS:	D	p. 182
31.	ANS:	C	p. 183
32.	ANS:	A	p. 182
33.	ANS:	E	p. 217
34.	ANS:	A	p. 219
35.	ANS:	A	p. 227
36.	ANS:	E	p. 223
37.	ANS:	C	p. 209
38.	ANS:	C	p. 209
39.	ANS:	E	p. 187
40.	ANS:	A	p. 228
41.	ANS:	B	p. 228
42.	ANS:	D	pp. 223–224
43.	ANS:	B	p. 225
44.	ANS:	C	p. 226
45.	ANS:	B	p. 240
46.	ANS:	B	p. 257
47.	ANS:	A	p. 257
48.	ANS:	D	p. 257
49.	ANS:	E	p. 261
50.	ANS:	C	p. 262

Unit 3 Test

Answer Section

Multiple Choice

1. ANS: B p. 288
2. ANS: A p. 290
3. ANS: C p. 300
4. ANS: D p. 304
5. ANS: C p. 310
6. ANS: E p. 326
7. ANS: B p. 331
8. ANS: E pp. 335–336
9. ANS: B p. 333
10. ANS: B p. 327
11. ANS: C p. 327
12. ANS: D p. 332
13. ANS: B p. 339
14. ANS: C p. 341
15. ANS: E p. 341
16. ANS: D p. 356
17. ANS: D p. 362
18. ANS: D p. 380
19. ANS: D p. 389
20. ANS: C p. 369
21. ANS: B p. 355, 363, 371, 377
22. ANS: D p. 415
23. ANS: A p. 415
24. ANS: C p. 418
25. ANS: A p. 411
26. ANS: B p. 412
27. ANS: C p. 418
28. ANS: E p. 444
29. ANS: C p. 448
30. ANS: A p. 453
31. ANS: D p. 466
32. ANS: D p. 469
33. ANS: A p. 476
34. ANS: B p. 441
35. ANS: A p. 446
36. ANS: E p. 446
37. ANS: C p. 448
38. ANS: B p. 467
39. ANS: D p. 479
40. ANS: D p. 514
41. ANS: A p. 499
42. ANS: A p. 507
43. ANS: A p. 516
44. ANS: D p. 521
45. ANS: C p. 523
46. ANS: B p. 522
47. ANS: C p. 502
48. ANS: D p. 511
49. ANS: B p. 513
50. ANS: E p. 525

Unit 4 Test

Answer Section

Multiple Choice

1. ANS: A p. 542
2. ANS: A p. 557
3. ANS: E p. 543
4. ANS: D p. 547
5. ANS: E p. 557
6. ANS: B p. 558
7. ANS: A p. 562
8. ANS: D p. 559
9. ANS: C p. 567
10. ANS: A p. 569
11. ANS: D p. 541
12. ANS: A p. 543
13. ANS: D pp. 546–547, 570
14. ANS: C p. 547
15. ANS: B p. 549
16. ANS: B p. 567
17. ANS: B pp. 555, 570
18. ANS: E p. 556
19. ANS: D pp. 566, 570
20. ANS: C p. 566–567
21. ANS: B p. 568
22. ANS: B p. 581
23. ANS: A p. 599
24. ANS: A p. 581
25. ANS: B p. 588
26. ANS: E p. 589
27. ANS: D p. 595
28. ANS: B p. 609
29. ANS: E p. 606
30. ANS: D p. 581–582
31. ANS: E p. 584
32. ANS: D p. 586
33. ANS: C p. 590
34. ANS: B pp. 593–594
35. ANS: C p. 597
36. ANS: D p. 598
37. ANS: D p. 610
38. ANS: C pp. 596, 610
39. ANS: E p. 602
40. ANS: B p. 605

Midterm Exam 1

Answer Section

Multiple Choice

1. ANS: A p. 12
2. ANS: D p. 17
3. ANS: E p. 13
4. ANS: D p. 12
5. ANS: A p. 26
6. ANS: C p. 29
7. ANS: C p. 26
8. ANS: A p. 28
9. ANS: C p. 34
10. ANS: E p. 44
11. ANS: C p. 43
12. ANS: E pp. 44–45
13. ANS: C p. 55
14. ANS: A pp. 62–63
15. ANS: A pp. 53, 63
16. ANS: A p. 72
17. ANS: D p. 73
18. ANS: C p. 73
19. ANS: B p. 86
20. ANS: A p. 79
21. ANS: D p. 84
22. ANS: A p. 90
23. ANS: E p. 104
24. ANS: D p. 123
25. ANS: B p. 108
26. ANS: E pp. 114, 128
27. ANS: D p. 100

28. ANS: B p. 137
29. ANS: E p. 162
30. ANS: B pp. 167–168
31. ANS: C p. 192
32. ANS: C p. 201
33. ANS: C p. 195
34. ANS: C p. 183
35. ANS: D p. 197
36. ANS: A p. 182
37. ANS: B p. 218
38. ANS: D p. 218
39. ANS: B p. 222
40. ANS: A p. 227
41. ANS: E p. 226
42. ANS: C p. 226
43. ANS: C p. 238
44. ANS: C pp. 240, 270
45. ANS: D p. 240
46. ANS: A p. 242
47. ANS: C p. 248
48. ANS: B p. 251
49. ANS: C p. 259
50. ANS: A p. 264

Midterm Exam 2

Answer Section

Multiple Choice

1. ANS: A p. 296
2. ANS: A p. 301
3. ANS: A p. 312
4. ANS: B p. 285
5. ANS: A p. 294
6. ANS: E p. 300–301
7. ANS: D p. 313
8. ANS: E p. 328
9. ANS: B p. 331
10. ANS: C p. 333
11. ANS: B p. 329
12. ANS: C p. 327
13. ANS: A p. 331
14. ANS: D p. 336
15. ANS: B p. 337
16. ANS: C p. 339
17. ANS: C p. 354
18. ANS: B p. 384
19. ANS: C p. 385
20. ANS: B p. 392
21. ANS: A p. 371
22. ANS: C p. 392
23. ANS: A p. 408
24. ANS: A p. 414
25. ANS: E p. 424
26. ANS: C p. 418
27. ANS: A p. 426
28. ANS: D p. 466
29. ANS: B p. 442
30. ANS: C p. 448
31. ANS: D p. 469
32. ANS: B p. 506
33. ANS: B p. 451
34. ANS: A p. 518
35. ANS: C p. 523
36. ANS: D p. 495
37. ANS: B p. 506
38. ANS: B pp. 509, 528
39. ANS: D p. 541
40. ANS: A p. 601
41. ANS: B p. 583
42. ANS: D p. 542
43. ANS: A p. 580
44. ANS: B p. 597
45. ANS: C p. 600
46. ANS: A pp. 579, 609
47. ANS: D p. 605
48. ANS: C p. 589
49. ANS: E p. 602
50. ANS: E p. 602

Final Exam

Answer Section

Multiple Choice

1. ANS: B p. 10
2. ANS: B p. 11
3. ANS: D p. 12
4. ANS: D p. 14
5. ANS: A p. 15
6. ANS: D p. 28
7. ANS: A pp. 30, 35
8. ANS: C p. 32
9. ANS: B p. 26
10. ANS: C p. 26
11. ANS: A p. 29
12. ANS: E p. 31
13. ANS: A p. 34
14. ANS: B p. 48
15. ANS: E p. 43
16. ANS: C p. 47
17. ANS: E p. 60
18. ANS: E pp. 29, 35
19. ANS: C p. 73
20. ANS: C pp. 30, 35
21. ANS: C p. 35
22. ANS: A p. 83
23. ANS: A p. 72
24. ANS: C p. 75
25. ANS: E p. 76
26. ANS: C p. 88
27. ANS: E p. 104
28. ANS: B p. 114
29. ANS: E p. 108
30. ANS: B p. 108
31. ANS: E p. 110
32. ANS: B p. 144
33. ANS: E p. 153
34. ANS: D p. 147
35. ANS: B p. 177
36. ANS: C p. 219
37. ANS: D p. 182
38. ANS: D p. 194
39. ANS: D p. 213
40. ANS: C p. 209
41. ANS: A p. 218
42. ANS: D p. 224
43. ANS: D p. 226
44. ANS: C p. 238
45. ANS: D p. 265
46. ANS: C pp. 247, 270
47. ANS: C p. 255
48. ANS: C p. 262
49. ANS: B p. 269

50. ANS: D p. 286
51. ANS: E p. 289
52. ANS: A p. 317
53. ANS: E p. 296
54. ANS: A p. 305
55. ANS: A p. 310
56. ANS: B p. 285
57. ANS: C p. 286
58 ANS: E p. 311
59. ANS: D p. 329
60. ANS: B p. 334
61. ANS: D p. 334
62. ANS: E p. 338
63. ANS: B p. 369
64. ANS: A p. 384
65. ANS: B p. 386
66. ANS: B p. 392
67. ANS: C p. 470
68. ANS: A p. 368
69. ANS: C p. 376
70. ANS: C p. 386
71. ANS: D p. 414
72. ANS: A p. 414
73. ANS: D p. 422
74. ANS: C p. 419
75. ANS: A p. 418
76. ANS: B p. 421
77. ANS: B p. 427
78. ANS: A p. 462
79. ANS: D p. 472
80. ANS: E p. 450
81. ANS: D p. 466
82. ANS: A p. 494
83. ANS: B p. 495
84. ANS: C p. 525
85. ANS: A p. 516
86. ANS: C p. 500
87. ANS: D p. 502
88. ANS: B p. 511
89. ANS: E p. 517
90. ANS: E p. 518
91. ANS: A pp. 566, 570
92. ANS: B p. 566
93. ANS: D p. 559
94. ANS: A p. 541
95. ANS: B p. 415
96. ANS: D p. 607
97. ANS: A p. 579
98. ANS: D p. 581–582
99. ANS: A p. 594
100. ANS: D p. 600